THE MIND'S EYE

Readings from
**SCIENTIFIC
AMERICAN**

THE MIND'S EYE

With Introductions by
Jeremy M. Wolfe
Massachusetts Institute of Technology

W. H. Freeman and Company
New York

Library of Congress Cataloging in Publication Data

Main entry under title:

The Mind's eye.

  "Readings from Scientific American."
  Bibliography: p.
  Includes index.
  1. Visual perception—Addresses, essays, lectures.
2. Vision—Physiological aspects—Addresses, essays,
lectures. I. Wolfe, Jeremy M. II. Scientific American.
BF241.M56 1986   153.7   85–16095
ISBN 0–7167–1767–0
ISBN 0–7167–1754–9 (pbk.)

Printed in the United States of America.

2 3 4 5 6 7 8 9 0   KP   4 3 2 1 0 8 9 8 7 6

CONTENTS

PREFACE

How do we see? About twenty-five years ago a famous professor at the Massachusetts Institute of Technology working in the field of artificial intelligence assigned the problem of duplicating human vision to one of his students as a summer project. After all, since computers had already begun to tackle such difficult problems as playing chess, surely the simple act of seeing could be mastered in one summer. Now, twenty-five years later, when computers can play a better game of chess than all but the best of the world's chess players, they still cannot see as well as a fish or a human infant.

Understanding vision is not a simple task. The seemingly effortless manner in which our visual system delivers a stable, colorful, three-dimensional perception of the world actually entails a great deal of very complicated and incompletely understood processing. Nevertheless, we do know a great deal about vision, more than about any of our other senses. The articles collected in this volume will take you on a tour through a number of different areas of vision research.

Visual processing can be divided into three basic steps:

$$\text{Reception} \rightarrow \text{extraction} \rightarrow \text{inference}$$

First, energy must be received from the outside world. Next, basic visual features are extracted from the input. Finally, on the basis of those extracted features, the visual system makes inferences about the visual world. Each section of this volume examines one of these levels of processing.

The first step of visual processing is to get external stimuli into the nervous system. We see "light," a narrow band of energy from the electromagnetic spectrum. At the back of the eye lies the retina, a collection of nerve cells that is, in fact, an extension of the brain. The optics of the eye form an upside-down image on the retina, and photosensitive cells convert electromagnetic energy into the electrochemical signals that are understood by the nervous system.

The human eye is admirably suited to the visual demands of human beings. Each of the articles in the first section of this book deals with a different set of eyes: fish, snakes, and insects. By studying the specific adaptations of their visual systems to their needs, we can examine the constraints that shaped the evolution of our own eyes.

The receptors in the retina give the nervous system a point-by-point assessment of the intensity of light. This input, further processed by other nerve cells in the retina, then moves down the optic nerve and into the brain. After an intermediate stop it arrives at the visual cortex, where we find cells that extract specific features of visual input. Where are there edges? What is moving? What is the size of the spot? What is the color? The articles in the second section discuss some of the evidence indicating that the visual system has special mechanisms to extract information about features such as color, motion, orientation, and size. It is this information that the "mind's eye" uses to create visual perception.

The word "create" is used quite deliberately in the previous sentence, for what we see is, indeed, a creation. The conclusion of most of the articles in the final section is that the visual system makes "inferences" about the world. These inferences are based on the features that the visual system has extracted from the input and also on perceptual rules. As an example of the creative nature of perception, consider the white page you are reading. If you are reading indoors, the light falling on the paper probably comes from an artificial source—an incandescent or fluorescent bulb. The light source is emitting wavelengths that are being reflected from the page and perceived by you as white. The black letters on the same page probably reflect about 5 percent as much light as does the white paper.

Suppose you take the book outdoors. Because the light level on a reasonably sunny day is far more than twenty times what it was indoors, the light reflected from the black letters outside is brighter than that reflected by the white page inside. Nevertheless, the letters remain perceptually black. Furthermore, the white page remains white, even though the wavelengths contained in sunlight are quite different from those in artificial light. The phenomena of brightness constancy and color constancy are simple demonstrations of the fact that you do not perceive physical features of visual stimulus. Instead, your perception is inferred from the stimulus.

Hermann von Helmholtz, the famous 19th century German scientist, wrote about the unconscious inferences made by our brains. I have followed his lead in calling the final step in visual perception "inference." However, it would be just as apt to call it "computation." The student who tried to make a seeing computer over the course of one summer has been joined by a host of researchers who are trying to understand the computations that are made automatically by our visual systems. Given edges and intensities, how do we determine the boundaries of objects? Given a two-dimensional image, how do we compute a three-dimensional perception?

The articles reprinted here will take you from the eye to the mind's eye. You will see that we know a great deal about vision and, I feel sure, you will understand why the problem was not dispensed with in a mere few weeks some twenty-five years ago.

Jeremy M. Wolfe
September 1985

I

EYES

I   EYES

INTRODUCTION

Light reception is the primary function of any visual system. The light we see, along with other forms of radiant energy such as X-rays or radio waves, is part of the electromagnetic (EM) spectrum. The difference between visible light and other parts of the EM spectrum is its wavelength (or energy—they are directly related). Waves of light are analogous to the waves that are formed when a pebble is tossed into a pool. The distance from the peak of one wave to the peak of the next is the wavelength. Visible light has wavelengths between about 400 and 700 nanometers (nm). A nanometer is 10^{-9}, or one-billionth, of a meter. For comparison, X-rays are around 10^{-10} meter long while radio waves are about 1 meter long. To our visual system, 400 nm looks violet. As wavelength increases, the perceived color of light changes through blue, to green, to yellow, orange, and, by the time we get above 600 nm, to red. We are bombarded by other wavelengths, but we do not see them.

Why then do we see only this narrow slice of the EM spectrum? The simplest answer is that our visual systems evolved in the light of the sun, and sunlight, by the time it reaches the surface of the earth, is strongest in the wavelengths between 400 and 700 nm. Human spectral sensitivity (sensitivity to different wavelengths) is well positioned to catch most of that light, although a fair amount of infrared radiation (700–1500 nm) and somewhat less ultraviolet radiation (250–400 nm) does reach the earth's surface, unseen by human eyes.

That this is not mere coincidence is elegantly illustrated in the article on color vision in fishes by Levine and MacNichol. They show that the spectral sensitivity of different species of fishes depends on the spectral distribution of light in the species' usual environment. Fishes living in muddy water have photoreceptors specialized for reddish brown colors. Those living in deep, blue water have photoreceptors for wavelengths at the blue-green end of the spectrum. There are even fishes with different spectral sensitivity in the upper and lower retina. Since the optics of the eye reverse the image, the upper retina receives input from below. In some fishes, this region is specialized for redder, muddier colors, while the lower retina, looking at the sky, is specialized for blue-green colors.

Whereas fishes living in restricted visual environments have restricted spectral sensitivities, some animals have sensitivities beyond ours. Newman and Hartline discuss one example—the infrared vision of certain types of snakes. Infrared radiation is a form of heat. It is not only found in sunlight but is emitted by all objects in proportion to their temperature. Thus, warm-blooded animals—of the sort that might make a good dinner for a snake—will be "brighter" than the background. In a snake the heat receptors that we all have in our skin are packed into the retinas of crude eyes that function in parallel with a snake's more standard eyes.

Newman and Hartline go on to show how some interactions between input from the infrared "pits" and the standard eyes are similar to the interactions between our own two eyes in normal binocular vision. For example, the snake's brain has cells that respond only when an object stimulates both the eye and the infrared pit. In my article on "hidden visual processes," I discuss mechanisms in human vision that respond only when both the left and the right eye are stimulated by the same thing.

Though they may differ in the details of spectral sensitivity, fishes, snakes, and humans all have eyes that are variations on the same basic theme—a single optical system forms an image on the retina.

The radically different eye of the insect is investigated in the article by Horridge. Insects have a compound eye in which each facet has a complete optical system of its own. Although the insect's eye is different from ours, there are certain similarities. For example, our vision is not uniformly good across the entire visual field. As you look at this sentence, you will notice that even though you can see a lot of surrounding space, you cannot see it very well. In fact, looking at this line, you cannot read a line a mere three lines up or down. On your retina there is a region, the fovea, where the photoreceptors are tightly packed, permitting very fine visual resolution. When you want to see something well, you move your eyes so that the image falls on the fovea. Some insects have the equivalent of a fovea in a region where many facets point in the same general direction. Others have two of these concentrations of facets in each eye, giving them, in effect, a second fovea.

Several basic points emerge from an examination of eyes and visual systems unlike our own. (1) The primary function of any visual system is reception. (2) The visual environment is different from species to species, and visual receptors have evolved accordingly. (3) There are basic principles of visual organization that transcend species. (4) Humans do not see the only visual world. We see our own visual world, which can be very different from the visual world of another species.

1

Color Vision in Fishes

by Joseph S. Levine and Edward F. MacNichol, Jr.
February 1982

The visual environments of fishes are blue, green or near infrared. The retinal pigments acquired by diverse fish species in adapting to these environments are a valuable clue to the evolution of the eye

The photosensitive cells of the retina are the outer extension of an animal's visual system. The cells catch the photons of visible light and in effect count them, thereby triggering a complex series of chemical and neural events that can result in visual sensation. In many animals the data-collecting function of the cells has developed to take advantage of discriminations possible on the basis of color as well as brightness, because in many environments color vision is an efficient means of gaining accurate information essential to survival. In deepwater environments, however, the number of photons that bathe an organism is much reduced and the color of the ambient light is confined to a narrow spectral band. The system of photoreceptor cells in the retina of a deep-water organism has correspondingly developed to maximize sensitivity to the available light rather than to provide color discrimination. Between the darkness at depth and the full sunlight at the surface there is a continuous range of luminous environments that vary in both color and intensity. In such a natural laboratory one encounters a wide variety of visual systems.

Several years ago we began an intensive study of the photoreceptors of teleost fishes (bony fishes, as opposed to cartilaginous ones such as sharks) in the hope of understanding how complex visual systems might have evolved from their precursors. The evolutionary reconstruction of the visual system cannot rely on fossil evidence because the soft tissues of the eye and the nerve pathways are not preserved. We chose therefore to investigate representatives from a variety of teleost families so that we could survey some of the relations among visual systems, visually dependent behavior and the environment. If the evolutionary relations among living teleost species are known on independent grounds, an examination of their visual systems and their visual ecology could lead to the reconstruction of the likely stages in the evolution of vision.

It might be supposed such a reconstruction would be relatively straightforward. One might assume, for example, that fishes known through fossil evidence to have undergone little recent evolutionary change would retain relatively primitive visual systems. Accordingly one might also assume that species evolving in relatively recent times would incorporate visual systems more advanced than the ones found in the older species. Both assumptions, however, take no account of the possibility that eyes may have evolved independently of other organs, because eyes themselves may confer selective advantages for such vital activities as finding food, avoiding predators and selecting a mate. The selective advantages of one visual system over another, in a particular environment for a particular behavioral repertory, may bring about changes in the eyes of a fish that is otherwise unaltered by evolutionary forces. The teleosts illustrate such evolutionary possibilities with particular clarity.

Explosive evolutionary radiation has emplaced between 17,000 and 30,000 species of teleosts in a broad range of aquatic habitats. Even single families of teleosts, with a wide variety of visually dependent types of behavior, occupy habitats that span nearly the full range of light zones in the sea and in freshwater lakes. Their eyes can differ so dramatically in size, shape, retinal organization and color sensitivity that one would never suspect, from examining the eyes alone, that the species are closely related. On the other hand, unrelated species inhabiting the same light zone can show remarkable similarities in their visual systems. For this reason primitive visual systems that may be preserved in living teleosts cannot be unequivocally distinguished from degenerate or specialized systems.

In spite of this difficulty, comparative ecological study can answer certain important evolutionary questions. What combination of selective advantages and operating constraints favors the possession of visual systems capable of discrimination over a broad range of colors and light intensities? Under what circumstances is the possession of such a complex system an encumbrance rather than an advantage? Although relatively little is known about the constraints on vision that are specifically related to feeding, fleeing or mating behavior, much has been learned about the lighting conditions that prevail underwater.

The solar radiation reaching the surface of the water is made up of photons of every visible wavelength, together with photons of the infrared and ultraviolet regions of the electromagnetic spectrum. The energies of visible-light photons correspond to colors or wavelengths, from violet with a wavelength of 400 nanometers to deep red with a wavelength of 700 nanometers. When light passes through the water, its intensity decreases, and the loss of intensity varies with color. Bodies of fresh water and salt water that do not contain much organic matter absorb violet and red light much more than they absorb light of intermediate wavelengths. Hence tropical oceans and clean lakes such as Crater Lake in Oregon and Lake Malawi in eastern Africa get bluer with depth as colors other than blue are absorbed. In such waters blue light can penetrate to a depth of more than 75 meters, whereas red and violet light are essentially absent below a depth of about 25 meters.

Unlike these "clear water" habitats, most Temperate Zone lakes, streams and coastal waters contain both yellow-green phytoplankton and dissolved organic matter from decaying plants and animals. In such waters light of all wavelengths is absorbed more strongly than it is in clear water, but the relative color intensities at each depth are quite different from what they are in clear water. The short-wavelength violet and blue light is the most strongly absorbed, and green or yellow-green light at wavelengths between 540 and 560 nanometers becomes increasingly dominant with depth. To the human eye the water looks green.

Marshes, swamps and "black water" rivers contain the same short-wave-

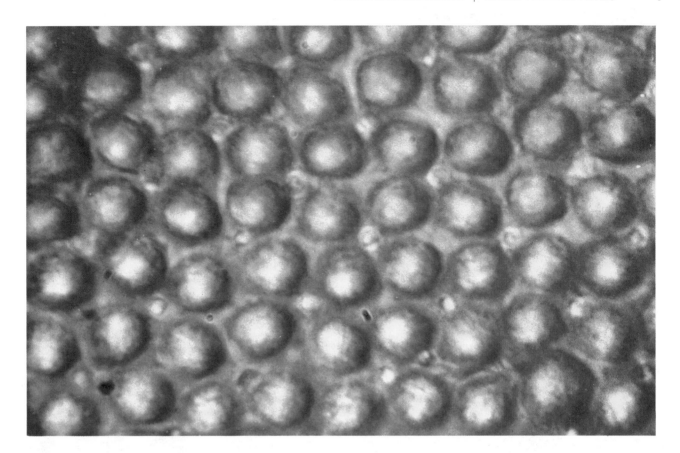

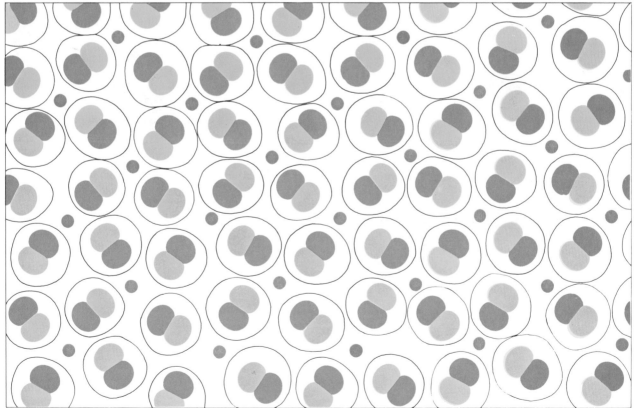

PHOTORECEPTOR CELLS in the retina of the black tetra fish (*Gymnocorymbus ternetzii*) form a regular mosaic pattern. In the photomicrograph at the top of the cone cells normally essential for color vision are shown as they appear from the back of the fish's retina, magnified 1,000 diameters. (Most of the rod cells, which are more sensitive to light than the cone cells, have been removed from the specimen for clarity.) Three kinds of cones are present in the retina of the black tetra: single cones holding a blue-sensitive visual pigment and double cones, made up of separate cells, holding both a green- and an orange-sensitive pigment. In the drawing at the bottom the color of the light that is maximally absorbed by each pigment is associated with the position of the pigments in the retina. The photomicrograph was made by the authors. The color of the cells in the photomicrograph is an artifact introduced by the technique of microscopy.

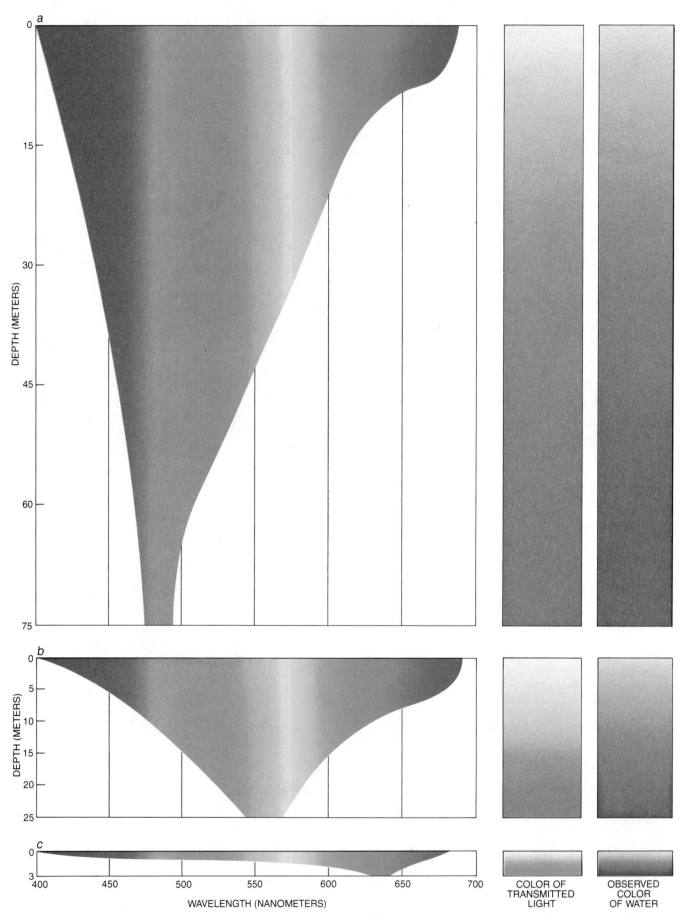

COLOR OF TRANSMITTED LIGHT

OBSERVED COLOR OF WATER

WAVELENGTH (NANOMETERS)

DEPTH (METERS)

TRANSMISSION OF LIGHT by water is dependent on the color or wavelength of the light. In clear oceans and lakes (*a*) the light becomes increasingly monochromatic and blue as its path length increases. In fresh water that carries green organic matter (*b*) light at all wavelengths is absorbed more quickly than it is in clear water, but the light becomes greener with path length. In rivers, swamps and marshes that carry large amounts of the products of plant and animal decay (*c*) absorption is rapid and the spectral distribution of the light shifts to the red. Such waters are called black because the human eye is relatively insensitive to light at long wavelengths; a less anthropomorphic name would be infrared water. The depths given for the maximum penetration of light are typical, but they vary widely.

absorbing compounds as lakes and streams, along with tannins, lignins and other products of more complete plant decomposition. The combined effects of the suspended and the dissolved matter can be the absorption of all light within about three meters of the surface; the maximally transmitted wavelength is 600 nanometers or longer, well into the red. To the eye such water usually appears dark or ruddy brown.

Light passing through water is also scattered in all directions by suspended particles and the water molecules themselves. When light is scattered, it must travel farther through the water to reach a given point; moreover, because of scattering every line of sight in the water is a source of photons, and so the water itself appears to be colored in all directions. This coloration is called background space light, and the combined effects of scattering and absorption cause it to vary with the direction of the line of sight.

Background space light has long been familiar to scuba divers, but it was not until the mid-1970's that spectro-radiometric measurements of it were made in tropical marine habitats. William N. McFarland of Cornell University and Frederick W. Munz of the University of Oregon quantitatively confirmed earlier observations that light along horizontal lines of sight is much more monochromatic than light along a vertical line of sight near the surface. McFarland and Munz recognized their finding as a major factor in the evolution of aquatic visual systems. Unlike terrestrial animals, which must distinguish food, predators and mates from whatever happens to be in the background at the time of sighting, fishes usually must detect objects against background space light that has a relatively constant color along any particular line of sight.

In the eye of a fish, as in the eye of a mammal, the photoreceptor cells onto which the incoming light is focused are filled with the photosensitive substances called visual pigments. Visual pigments were independently discovered in 1877 by the German physiologists Franz Boll and Wilhelm Friedrich Kühne. Boll noted that when a frog's retina is removed from the eye, it is initially bright red but bleaches in light, becoming first yellow and finally colorless. Kühne found soon afterward that the pigment in the rod cells (the rod-shaped photoreceptor cells) of many animals is also red and bleaches when it is exposed to light. In a living animal the color of the pigment is restored if the animal is placed in the dark, but in cells that have been removed from the animal the bleaching of the pigment is permanent.

The visual pigments catch photons of light by absorbing them, just as water does. To appreciate the importance of

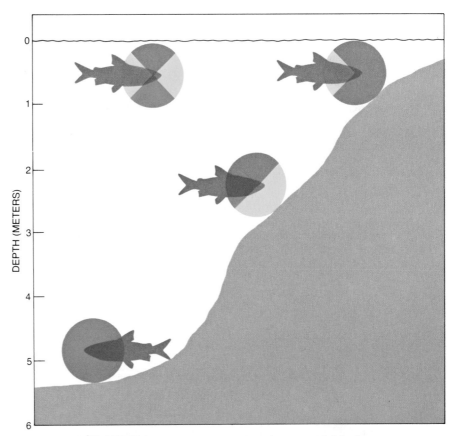

SCATTERING OF LIGHT by water molecules and particles suspended in the water causes the dominant color of the transmitted light to vary with the direction of the line of sight. Because every point on every line of sight is a source of photons the water itself appears to be differently colored in all directions. The coloration imposes a background of space light against which any object must be viewed, and it also interposes a veiling brightness between the observer and the object. The illustration shows how the coloration varies with direction in four microhabitats of a "black water" river: at the surface and on the bottom in shallow and in deep water.

the pigments, however, it is necessary to consider the wavelengths of light that are maximally absorbed rather than those that are maximally transmitted. The pigment in human rod cells, for example, is pink, hence the name rhodopsin, from the Greek words meaning "rose" and "vision." Rhodopsin appears pink because it transmits red and blue light, whereas its absorption maximum is at a wavelength of 500 nanometers, in the blue-green region of the spectrum.

When a visual pigment absorbs photons, the molecules in the pigment undergo structural changes and trigger electrochemical responses in the photoreceptor cells that hold the pigment. The response of each cell is determined in part by the number of photons absorbed by the pigment but not by the wavelengths of the photons; once a photon is absorbed its wavelength no longer affects the output of the photoreceptor cell. The only means the visual system has of extracting information about the color of incident light is to take into account the statistical probability that one of its pigments will absorb a photon with a given wavelength.

How can one determine these absorption probabilities? Early investigators extracted pigments chemically from a whole eye, and so their investigations

were limited almost entirely to the pigments in the rod cells. Rod pigments are more abundant and easier to extract than the pigments in cone cells (the cone-shaped photoreceptor cells found in many retinas). After a rod pigment was extracted its spectrum was analyzed by a spectrophotometer. In the instrument a beam of monochromatic light of selected visible wavelengths was passed through the pigment and the intensity of the transmitted light was measured. The measured intensity was compared with the intensity of a reference beam from the same source that did not pass through the pigment. It is possible to transform the data mathematically into a graph that shows the optical density of the pigment as a function of wavelength; the graph is called an absorbance spectrum. One can also calculate the probability that a visual pigment will absorb a photon of a given wavelength from the absorbance spectrum of the pigment.

The method we employ to determine the absorbance spectra of visual pigments is conceptually identical with the method described above, except that we are able to record the spectra of pigments in individual photoreceptor cells. The instrument we use is the microspectrophotometer, a spectrophotometer that incorporates a high-powered microscope so that a magnified area of the image of the specimen can be spectrally analyzed. Such instruments are available in fewer than a dozen laboratories throughout the world. Earlier versions of the microspectrophotometer in our laboratory were developed by William B. Marks of Johns Hopkins University and one of us (MacNichol) in the early 1960's and by Ferenc I. Hárosi of the National Institute of Neurological Diseases and Stroke in the early 1970's. The instrument enables us to examine not only the different pigments in different kinds of photoreceptor cells but also the distribution of the cells in the retina.

To prepare a retinal specimen for microspectrophotometry the thin layer of photoreceptor cells must be separated from the pigment epithelium, a layer of retinal tissue behind the cells that absorbs stray light in the eye. This is accomplished first by soaking the retina in a saline solution and then teasing the layers apart surgically. The layer of photoreceptor cells is mounted on a thin microscope cover glass, and a second cover glass is placed over the cells in such a way as to flatten them on the first glass. All the work must be done in the dark or under infrared illumination, since otherwise the pigments in the specimen would bleach and so be of no use for getting spectral data. Hence in order to position the slide and focus the image of the specimen for scanning by the microspectrophotometer we employ infrared illumination at a wavelength that is not appreciably absorbed by any visual pigment. We observe the specimen on a television monitor connected to an infrared-sensitive television camera, which receives an image of the specimen magnified 1,000 diameters.

Once a photoreceptor cell has been aligned with the path of the scanning beam of the microspectrophotometer the recording of the absorbance spectrum is virtually automatic. A low-intensity, monochromatic beam of light is passed through the apparatus, first without the specimen cell and then with the specimen cell in place. The intensities of the two transmitted beams for each wavelength are recorded by a small

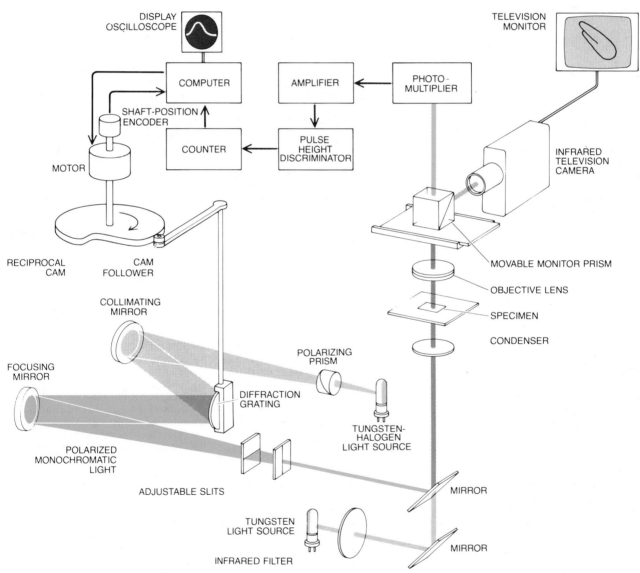

MICROSPECTROPHOTOMETER determines the absorbance spectrum for the visual pigment in a single photoreceptor cell. The apparatus measures the ratio of the intensity of a beam of monochromatic light that passes through the pigment to the intensity of an identical beam that does not pass through the pigment. In the schematic diagram each beam is polarized and then split into its spectral components by a diffraction grating. The wavelength of the monochromatic beam is calibrated to the position of a camshaft that controls the grating. Hence the precise wavelength of the input beam and the intensity of the output can be registered simultaneously in a computer. The pigments will bleach and lose their ability to absorb light if they are exposed to bright light. Therefore the beams passing through the specimens are held to low intensity, and the individual photons in the beam are converted into electric pulses by a photomultiplier. The pulses are then amplified, sorted from spurious random signals and tallied in a counter, whose output is periodically read into a computer. To position and focus the specimens infrared illumination is used in combination with an infrared television camera and monitor.

computer and compared. By working with low-intensity beams and by scanning the spectrum rapidly and repetitively we avoid having to compensate for the bleaching of the pigment every time the light passes through the specimen cell.

Almost all visual pigments absorb light of all visible wavelengths to some degree. Each pigment, however, has a well-defined wavelength for which the absorption probability is maximized, and the probabilities fall off rather sharply for both longer and shorter wavelengths. A deepwater fish with only one visual pigment would have the highest possible visual sensitivity if the maximum absorption probability of the pigment were matched to the color of the background space light. One of the earliest successes of visual ecology was establishing that in nonmigratory, deepwater marine fishes such matches are common. The light available to fishes more than 100 meters down is both dim and blue, at wavelengths between 470 and 490 nanometers. The maximum absorption wavelengths of the rod pigments closely fit the spectral distribution of the ambient light.

The rod pigments of coastal marine and freshwater species do not, however, follow the spectral distribution of available light as closely as those of deepwater species. The rods of Temperate Zone fishes whose habitat is shallow salt water are most sensitive to blue-green light with wavelengths between 500 and 510 nanometers, even though the local space light is yellow-green at wavelengths between 525 and 550 nanometers. Rod pigments in freshwater fishes from both deep and medium-depth habitats appear to be limited to a maximum absorption probability at wavelengths no longer than 540 nanometers, even though reddish orange light with a wavelength of 600 nanometers dominates the space light in their environment.

In 1966 J. N. Lythgoe of the University of Sussex suggested that the apparently mismatched pigments were set off from the color of the space light in order to maximize visual contrast. Lythgoe pointed out that when a pigment is matched to the space light, there is a relatively high contrast between a dark object, which deposits relatively few photons on the visual pigment, and the space light, which deposits many photons. A bright object, however, will deposit many photons on the pigment no matter what its color, and so it will not be strongly distinguished from the background space light. On the other hand, if the light illuminating the object is spectrally broad and the pigment is not matched to the space light, the situation will be reversed. A dark object and the space light will both appear dark, so that they will be relatively indistinguishable. A bright object will look bright, how-

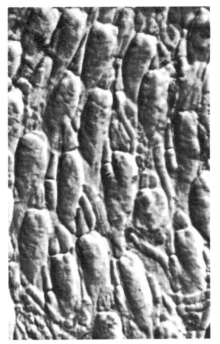
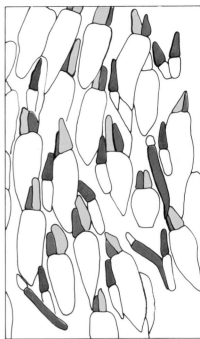

CONE CELLS of the black tetra, here magnified 500 diameters, differ according to shape as well as pigment content. Three kinds of cones are visible: large double cones, composed of separate cells, which carry the orange- and the green-sensitive pigments, and the smaller single cones, which carry the blue-sensitive pigment. A few long rod cells can also be seen; in the black tetra rods are maximally sensitive to green light. The photomicrograph was made by flattening the cells shown end on in the top illustration on page 5. The cells must be held flat between two cover glasses before the absorbance spectra can be made. In the diagram the position of the pigments in the cells is indicated by the colors to which they are maximally sensitive.

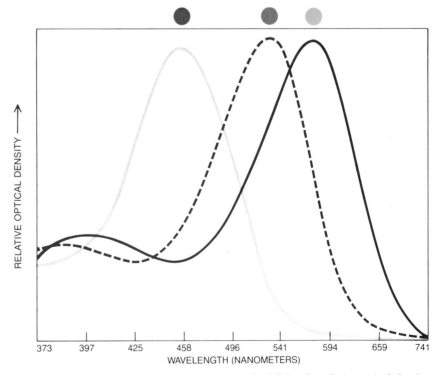

ABSORBANCE SPECTRA show, for each wavelength of light, the relative optical density of a visual pigment; they can be related mathematically to the probability that a photon of that wavelength will be absorbed by a visual pigment. Three absorbance spectra, one spectrum for each pigment of the cichlid fish (*Cichlasoma longimanus*), are graphed. The colors at the top of each curve indicate the appearance to the human visual system of the wavelengths of light to which each pigment is maximally sensitive, at 455, 532 and 579 nanometers respectively. For convenience in analysis the machine employed by the authors plots the absorbance of the pigments as a function of frequency. Hence when the same curves are employed to represent absorbance as a function of wavelength, the wavelength increments vary along the horizontal axis.

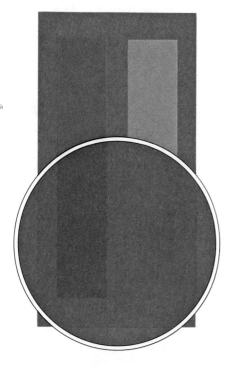

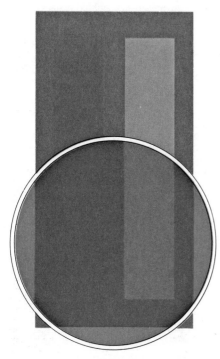

MULTIPLE-PIGMENT visual systems in fishes may initially have evolved because they enhanced the contrast of light and dark objects with the space light rather than because they were helpful in discriminating hue. For a monochromat whose blue-sensitive visual pigment matches the blue space light found in open-water marine habitats (*upper illustration*) a dark object is clearly visible against the background, but a light object is nearly invisible. A green-sensitive visual pigment that does not match the background (*lower illustration*) provides contrast between a light object and the background, although a dark object is nearly invisible. Fishes that incorporate both pigments can distinguish light and dark objects in their environment, even though they may lack the neural interconnections necessary to discriminate solely on the basis of hue.

ever, and so now it will be strongly distinguished from the space light [*see illustration at left*].

The rod cells are specially adapted for low-intensity illumination. Since in a given species they usually contain only one kind of pigment, vision that must depend on rods is responsive only to variations of light intensity. To a fish with rod cells only (a rod monochromat) the world looks as though it were photographed on black and white film through a color filter. Dark blue objects are indistinguishable from dark red or dark green ones, and bright colors are easily confused with white.

Nevertheless, a monochromat can conform its behavior to take maximum advantage of the contrast between the space light and relatively dark objects. For example, the skipjack tuna (*Katsuwonus pelamis*) appears to carry only one visual pigment, even though it possesses both rods and cones. Munz and McFarland noted that the skipjack maneuvers so that it can rush up to attack its prey from below. Viewed from below the prey is silhouetted against vertical space light, and the skipjack, whose single-pigment sensitivity is matched to the space light, can exploit the contrast between its relatively dark prey and the relatively bright space light.

Many fishes, however, have two or three classes of cone cells in addition to their rod cells. Each class of cones is usually associated with a particular visual pigment, and microspectrophotometric measurements have shown that rod and cone pigments have approximately equal probabilities of absorbing photons. Nevertheless, because of differences among rods and cones and the nature of their interactions with other cells in the retina, activating cone vision requires light much more intense than that required to activate rod vision. Cones are generally associated with color vision, and the discrimination of colors bestows a clear evolutionary advantage in habitats where light is bright and made up of many colors. Individual cone cells, however, can distinguish colors no better than rod cells: their output too depends on the number of photons absorbed by their pigments but not on the wavelengths of the photons. Even when several kinds of pigment are present in the photoreceptor cells in the retina, additional neural "wiring" is required before discriminations can be made solely on the basis of color. Hence it is likely that the evolutionary advantages initially conferred by the cones were not directly related to color vision. The advantages of the cones probably derived instead from their better adaptation to bright light and from the fact that a multiple-pigment visual system makes visual contrast possible across a broader spectral band than a single-pigment system does.

Some saltwater fishes that live near the surface, such as the mahimahi (*Coryphaena hippurus*), have two different cone pigments, one that absorbs mostly in the green and one that absorbs mostly in the blue. Such a dichromatic visual system is sensitive to light across a broader spectral band than a monochromatic system is, simply because more pigments give rise to efficient absorption

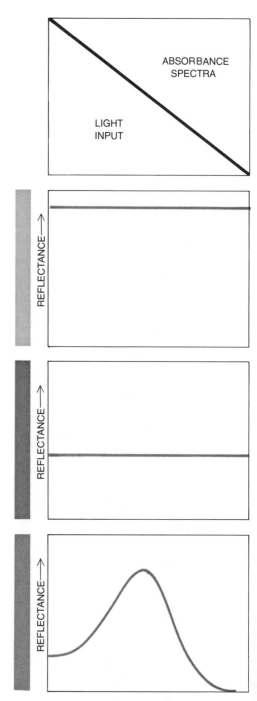

RESPONSE of a photoreceptor cell to a visual stimulus depends on the intensity of the stimulus and on the filter characteristics of the absorbing pigment. The wavelength of an incoming photon is irrelevant to the output of the cell once the photon has been absorbed.

in more regions of the spectrum. When a saltwater dichromat looks upward, the green pigment is well matched to the space light, whereas when it looks forward or downward the blue pigment is the better match.

McFarland and Munz have contended, however, that from an evolutionary standpoint the major advantage of two-pigment visual systems over one-pigment ones is that two-pigment systems allow both dark and bright objects to be discriminated against the background space light. When a blue-and-green-sensitive dichromat looks upward, the green-absorbing pigment enables the fish to distinguish dark objects against the predominantly green space light; the blue-absorbing pigment allows bright objects to be differentiated. When the fish looks forward or downward, the roles of the two pigments are reversed, but the net effect remains that both bright and dark objects can be distinguished against the background.

Our data show that the cone pigments of teleost fishes correspond rather well to the illumination available in the fishes' local environment. The broadest range of visual pigments is found among

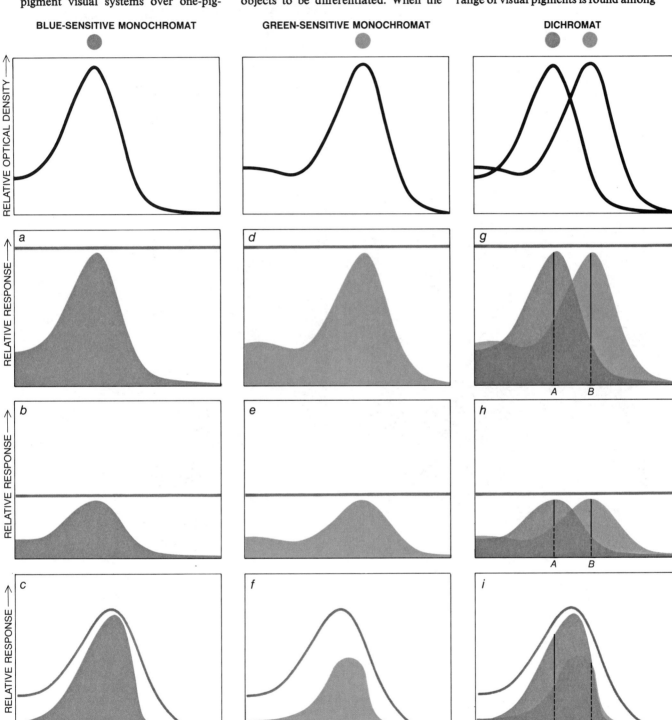

The table shows how the output of the cells (*areas shaded in blue and green*) varies with the input of the three colors shown in the illustration at the left. The output of the blue-sensitive cones is similar for the light gray and the blue inputs (*a, c*). Dark gray areas give reduced output (*b*), so that they would contrast with the background for a blue-sensitive monochromat. The output of the green-sensitive cones, on the other hand, is similar for the dark gray and the blue inputs (*e, f*), whereas the output for the light gray input (*d*) contrasts with the background. A dichromatic pigment system can also be the basis of color vision (*g, h, i*). A cell that monitors differences between the outputs of the two kinds of cones would distinguish light at wavelength *A* from light at *B*, no matter what the intensity of the light.

DAYLIGHT

CREPUSCULAR

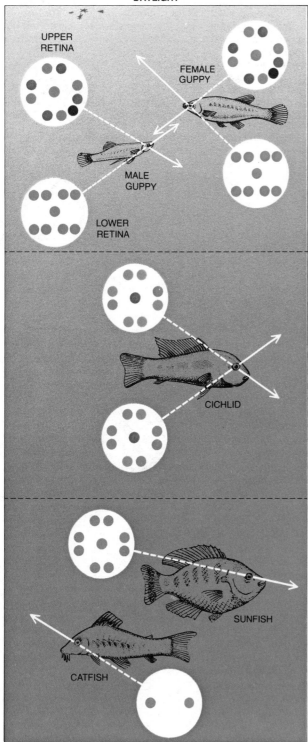

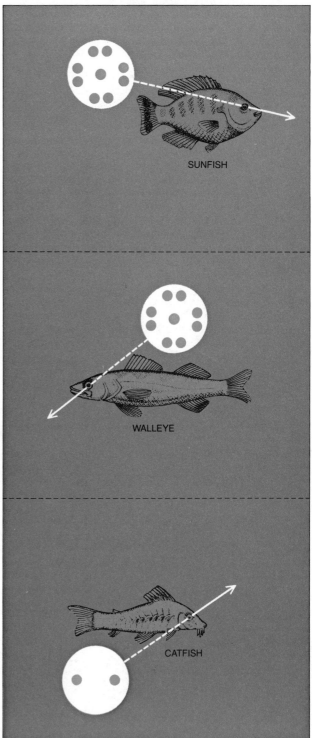

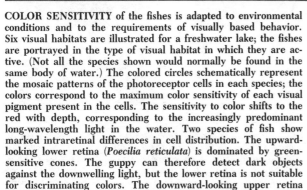

COLOR SENSITIVITY of the fishes is adapted to environmental conditions and to the requirements of visually based behavior. Six visual habitats are illustrated for a freshwater lake; the fishes are portrayed in the type of visual habitat in which they are active. (Not all the species shown would normally be found in the same body of water.) The colored circles schematically represent the mosaic patterns of the photoreceptor cells in each species; the colors correspond to the maximum color sensitivity of each visual pigment present in the cells. The sensitivity to color shifts to the red with depth, corresponding to the increasingly predominant long-wavelength light in the water. Two species of fish show marked intraretinal differences in cell distribution. The upward-looking lower retina (*Poecilia reticulata*) is dominated by green-sensitive cones. The guppy can therefore detect dark objects against the downwelling light, but the lower retina is not suitable for discriminating colors. The downward-looking upper retina is made up of all three types of cone and is therefore sensitive to a broad spectrum of colors. In mating displays the male guppy takes a position below or in front of the female so that his colors will be registered on the most color-sensitive area of the female's retina. The upward-looking lower retina of the cichlid is also primarily sensitive to middle-wavelength radiation, whereas its downward-looking upper retina is more sensitive to long-wavelength light. The differences correspond to the spectral distribution of the background space light along different lines of sight and to the variations among the visual tasks each species must perform. The retinal mosaic patterns of the sunfish (*Lepomis macrochirus*), the catfish (*Corydoras meyers*) and the walleye (*Stizostedion vitreum*) are all relatively uniform. The sunfish feeds on phytoplankton near the surface at dusk or dawn and follows the plankton downward during the day, so that the fish is active in visually similar environments throughout most of the day.

species that are active near the surface, where the light is bright and spectrally broad. In salt water at intermediate depths the red, long-wavelength light from the surface is almost entirely absorbed, and at such depths most saltwater species lack pigments that absorb red light. Their cones are maximally sensitive to blue and green light.

One exception to this trend is the sea raven (*Hemitripterus americanus*), which we studied with Hárosi and Barbara-Ann Collins of the Marine Biological Laboratory at Woods Hole, Mass. Sea ravens possess three pigments, maximally sensitive to blue, green and yellow-green light, which cover a much broader spectral range than one would expect in a fish that spends most of its life at depths of more than 100 meters. To understand the adaptive utility of a fish's visual system, however, one must consider the fish's total behavioral repertory. In the sea raven's breeding season, which is in late fall, the fish moves to shallow water and thus to brighter and spectrally broader light. The bodies of reproductive individuals turn bright yellow, orange and scarlet, and after fertilization the eggs are deposited on a species of sponge that is colored bright orange or yellow. Such behavior requires visual discriminations in the middle- to long-wavelength regions of the spectrum and so calls for a wide range of visual pigments.

In most freshwater habitats the utility of blue-sensitive cones diminishes with depth because the transmitted light from the surface is red-shifted instead of blue-shifted. The visual systems of the freshwater fishes we examined can be divided into four groups, based on the maximum absorption sensitivity of their visual pigments and on the physical appearance of their photoreceptor cells. In the first group are fishes such as the guppy (*Poecilia reticulata*) and the giant danio (*Danio malabaricus*), which confine themselves to the region directly below the surface. Their visual systems are similar to those of shallow-depth marine species; they are characterized by three visual pigments, maximally sensitive in the violet, the blue-green and the yellow-green.

The retinal sensitivity of the guppy is closely linked to its behavior patterns. The upper retina, onto which is focused light from below and in front of the guppy's visual field, is a mosaic of cone cells sensitive to three widely spaced spectral regions; it is well designed to make color discriminations. The lower retina, however, onto which is focused light from above the visual field, is lined with cells that all contain the same green-sensitive pigment. John A. Endler of the University of Utah noted recently that when male guppies display their conspicuous coloration in an effort to attract females, they do so from a position ahead of and

slightly below the object of their desire. Such a position in the visual field of the female ensures that the image of the male falls on the most color-sensitive region of the female's retina. The green-sensitive lower retina is best suited to finding dark bits of food silhouetted against the predominantly green vertical space light.

The second group of freshwater fishes also have three kinds of visual pigment, but their maximum sensitivities lie in longer-wavelength regions of the spectrum than those of the pigments in the first group. Such fishes include the tiger barb (*Barbus tetrazona*) and the cichlid fish (*Cichlasoma longimanus*); their sensitivity to long-wavelength light is an apparent evolutionary response to the rapid loss of short-wavelength light in the heavily stained waters they inhabit.

The bluegill (*Lepomis macrochirus*), the walleye (*Stizostedion vitreum*), the piranha (*Serrasalmus* sp.) and other fishes in the third group have few if any blue-sensitive cells in their retinas, although they do have green- and red-sensitive cells. They are active primarily at dawn or dusk near the surface, although many species feed in deeper parts of the water column during the day. Hence their spectral environment remains roughly the same throughout their active period. The red-sensitive pigments of these fishes make them far more sensitive to long-wavelength radiation than human beings are. The so-called black water inhabited by many such fishes is actually illuminated with near-infrared space light that is visible to them.

The retinas of the species in the fourth group are made up entirely of rods and green- and red-sensitive cones. No blue-sensitive pigments have been found in these cones, and in some species green-sensitive pigments seem to be missing as well. The fishes probably retain red-sensitive cones only because the dim background space light is highly red-shifted; otherwise they would probably be rod monochromats. The species in the group include numerous catfishes (such as *Corydoras meyers*) and the ecologically similar red-tailed black shark (*Labeo bicolor*).

It is likely that color vision, the ability to distinguish light on the basis of wavelength as well as intensity, evolved some time after two-pigment visual systems were in place. To be capable of color vision a fish not only must have two or more visual pigments whose absorbance spectra overlap; it also must have neural interconnections that can compare the signals of the photoreceptors in an appropriate way. To understand how this is accomplished consider the effect of a monochromatic red stimulus at a wavelength of 630 nanometers on the eye of a cichlid. The cichlid's eye has three visual pigments, including a yellow-absorbing pigment at a wave-

length of 579 nanometers and a green-absorbing one at 532 nanometers. No matter what the intensity of the red stimulus, the yellow-absorbing pigment will absorb more of the red photons than the green-absorbing pigment. On the other hand, a yellow-green stimulus at a wavelength of 540 nanometers will have approximately the same effect on the yellow-absorbing pigment that it has on the green-absorbing one, no matter what the light intensity of the stimulus is.

The output of a nerve cell that monitors both kinds of photoreceptor cell can be dependent on the difference between the two incoming signals. Such a cell would enable the cichlid to distinguish red from yellow-green, even though the brightness of the two colors as measured by one class of the cichlid's cone cells might be identical. Cells that process signals from photoreceptors of different classes were first discovered in fish retinas by the Swedish physiologist Gunnar Svaetichin and one of us (MacNichol) in the 1950's. They are called color-opponent cells, and they have been found at several levels of the visual system of many species.

Since color-opponent cells depend on the difference between photoreceptor signals, the discrimination of hue is most accurate in regions of the spectrum where the absorbance spectra of at least two visual pigments overlap and exhibit markedly different slopes. If the absorbance spectra have the same slope or if they do not overlap, the difference in output of the two associated classes of photoreceptors is a constant and hue discrimination is poor. The addition of a third pigment or even a fourth to a visual system, together with the appropriate color-opponent cells, can make hue discrimination possible in such "dead" spectral regions. Of course, a third or fourth pigment can also support the absolute sensitivity of a visual system to an even wider band of wavelengths than two pigments can.

Given the evolutionary advantages of hue discrimination over the ability merely to distinguish the intensity of light, why is color vision not universal among teleosts? For a hue-sensitive retina to function properly it must be bathed in enough light over a broad band of wavelengths to stimulate substantial signals from all types of cones. Any photoreceptor cells that do not emit signals leave "holes" in the visual image. Holes degrade the image, and so any cone pigments in the retina that do not contribute frequently to the visual image are actually dysfunctional. A fish that is active only at night or at twilight, or one that lives in the deep sea, seldom encounters enough light to stimulate cone cells at all. For such a fish, and apparently for many of man's primate relatives, the price of survival in the dark is the loss of sensitivity to color.

2

The Infrared "Vision" of Snakes

by Eric A. Newman and Peter H. Hartline
March 1982

Snakes of two families can detect and localize sources of infrared radiation. Infrared and visible-light information are integrated in the brain to yield a unique wide-spectrum picture of the world

Rattlesnakes can strike accurately even at night when darkness hides their prey. The strike is guided by heat: infrared radiation emitted by the warm-blooded target. The radiation is sensed by an extraordinary system that enables rattlesnakes to "see" in a region of the electromagnetic spectrum where animals generate their own radiant energy.

The infrared "eyes" of the rattlesnake are the pit organs, a pair of deep cavities in the head that open on the side of the head below and in front of the eyes. The pit organs are richly supplied with heat-sensitive nerve fibers connected to the brain. All snakes of the subfamily Crotalinae, the pit vipers, have pit organs and are sensitive to infrared radiation. In North America these snakes include the cottonmouth (water moccasin) and the copperhead as well as the rattlesnake. Pythons and many other members of the family Boidae (boid snakes), distant relatives of the pit vipers, also have heat-sensitive pits. In contrast to the pit vipers, they have many pits on the scales bordering their mouth, as many as 13 pairs.

Infrared sensitivity in pit vipers and boid snakes has apparently evolved from the somatic sensory system. In man and other mammals this sensory system is concerned with the sensations of, among other things, touch, pressure, temperature and pain. In mammals sensory messages are conducted from the facial area to the brain by the trigeminal nerve. In infrared-sensitive snakes a substantial part of the trigeminal nerve is devoted to the pit organs and infrared sensitivity. In the course of evolution the somatic sensory system of pit vipers and boids has developed into a sense much like vision. Pit vipers and boid snakes have also evolved specialized nuclei, or clusters of nerve-cell bodies, in the brain to receive and process the sensory information coming from the pit organs. The nuclei relay information to the optic tectum of the midbrain, a structure known for its role in vision and in the spatial representation of sensory information.

Like other animals, human beings learn to associate several sensory modalities with real objects of many kinds. For example, both the sight of a bird and the sound of its song help to localize and identify it. In an analogous way the optic tectum of infrared-sensitive snakes combines infrared signals from the pit organs with visual signals from the eyes. The integration of visual and infrared information in the tectum gives pit vipers and boid snakes a unique view of the world, a view that compares and contrasts visual and infrared images.

Although the infrared pit organs were described long ago by anatomists, their function remained obscure until the 1930's, when G. Kingsley Noble and A. Schmidt of the American Museum of Natural History in New York showed that the pits detect heat. They found that rattlesnakes could differentiate between a warm light bulb (covered with an opaque cloth) and a cold one. Snakes oriented and struck toward warm bulbs as long as their pits remained uncovered. They ignored all bulbs, warm as well as cold, if the pits were blocked.

In the 1950's Theodore H. Bullock and his colleagues at the University of California at Los Angeles demonstrated that the pit organ functions by sensing the infrared radiation given off by warm objects. These investigators monitored the nerve impulses in the axons (long nerve-cell fibers) of the trigeminal nerve that are connected to the pit. They found that impulses are triggered equally well by a warm object whether it is presented to a rattlesnake in the light or in a totally dark room. The axons do not respond, even in a lighted room, if the pit is exposed to the same object once it has cooled. Furthermore, the axon's activity in response to a warm object vanishes if a heat-absorbing glass filter is inserted between the pit and the object, even though the glass lets through nearly all the visible light. In the complementary experiment, where a filter was inserted that let through no visible radiation but passed most of the infrared, the response was only slightly reduced. Thus it was conclusively demonstrated that the pit organ is sensitive to radiation at infrared wavelengths.

Just how good is the rattlesnake's infrared sense? How accurately can a rattlesnake localize a warm object? How sensitive are the infrared detectors? Answers to these questions have come from a combination of behavioral and neurophysiological experiments.

In order to determine how accurately a rattlesnake can localize a warm object Laurence R. Stanford and Michael S. Loop, working with one of us (Hartline) at the University of Illinois at Urbana-Champaign, measured the striking accuracy of blindfolded snakes. A rattlesnake whose eyes (but not its pits) had been occluded with blinders was put on a raised pedestal in the middle of a circular enclosure. An infrared source (the heated tip of a soldering iron) was then presented to the snake just beyond its striking range. An experimenter introduced the soldering iron at various angles from zero to 60 degrees to the left or right of where the snake was facing. A video camera was ready to record the expected strike; the accuracy of the strike would be measured from the videotape.

The snakes refused to cooperate; they almost never struck toward the soldering iron. Apparently the stimulus was not sufficiently meaningful to them. The somewhat diabolical solution was to give the snake a mild electric shock just before each presentation of the soldering iron. The snakes now struck often enough so that we could measure the accuracy of their response. Even with both eyes securely covered the strikes were accurate to within about five degrees of dead center, regardless of whether the target originally lay straight ahead or off to the side. That is very impressive, and for a mouse it is deadly.

How can an investigator measure the sensitivity of the infrared sense? Bullock's method was to record the frequency of action potentials, or nerve impulses, in the trigeminal-nerve axons leading away from the pit organ. This neurophysiological approach can give an indication of the ultimate sensitivity

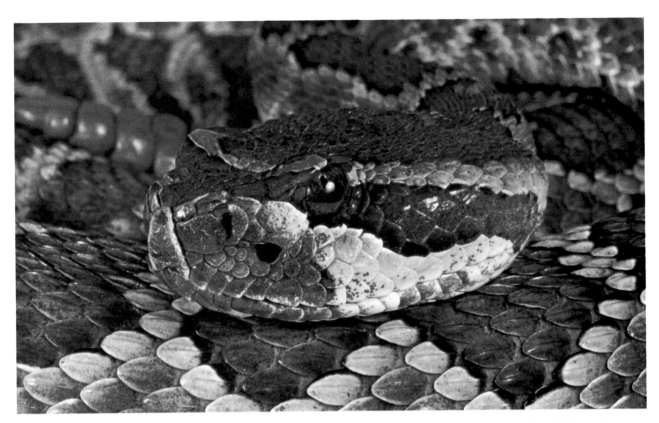

SOUTHERN PACIFIC RATTLESNAKE, a native of the western U.S., can locate weak sources of infrared radiation by means of its pit organs, a pair of cavities in front of and under its eyes. In rattlesnakes and other members of the pit-viper family the radiation is detected by an extremely thin heat-sensitive membrane that stretches across the back of each pit. The field of view of each pit extends from about 25 degrees beyond the animal's midline to 105 degrees at the side and from 45 degrees below the horizontal to 60 degrees above it.

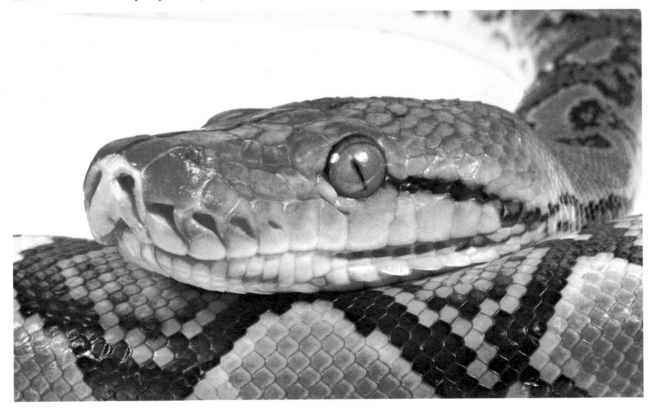

RETICULATED PYTHON, a native of southern Asia, has 13 pairs of pits in the scales above and below its mouth. This photograph shows five pits on the left side of the snout and one on the right. Six other pits border the lower lip, below and behind the eye. Other boid snakes (snakes of the family Boidae), including the tree boas, have similar arrays of pits. The back surface of each pit is highly sensitive to heat energy. Each pit has a slightly different field of view. Still other boid snakes, including the boa constrictors, do not have discrete pits but have infrared-sensitive scales on their face. Both of the photographs on this page were made by one of the authors (Newman).

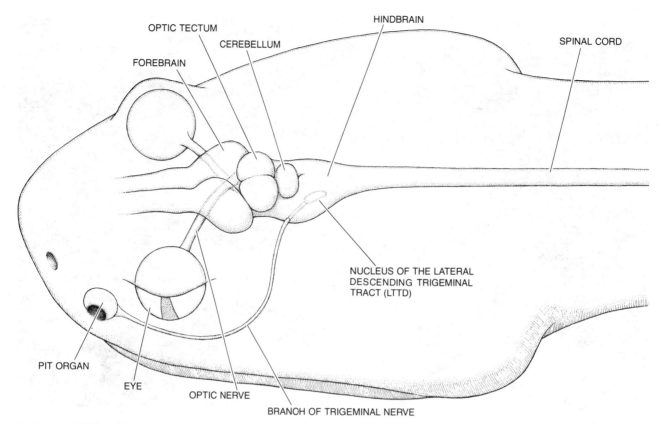

FOREBRAIN

OPTIC TECTUM

CEREBELLUM

HINDBRAIN

SPINAL CORD

NUCLEUS OF THE LATERAL
DESCENDING TRIGEMINAL
TRACT (LTTD)

PIT ORGAN

EYE

OPTIC NERVE

BRANCH OF TRIGEMINAL NERVE

STRUCTURES IN THE BRAIN and the nerve pathways associated with the infrared sensory system of pit vipers have only recently been worked out. A principal puzzle, now solved, was how the information gathered by the pit organ and carried by impulses in the trigeminal nerve finds its way to the optic tectum, a midbrain structure that plays a prominent role in the processing of visual information.

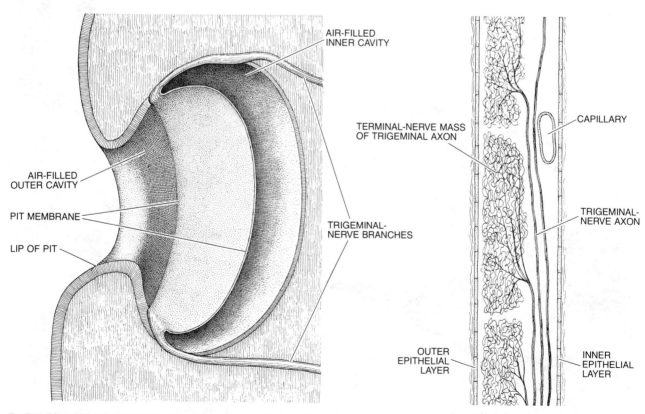

AIR-FILLED
INNER CAVITY

AIR-FILLED
OUTER CAVITY

PIT MEMBRANE

LIP OF PIT

TRIGEMINAL-
NERVE BRANCHES

TERMINAL-NERVE MASS
OF TRIGEMINAL AXON

CAPILLARY

TRIGEMINAL-
NERVE AXON

OUTER
EPITHELIAL
LAYER

INNER
EPITHELIAL
LAYER

RATTLESNAKE PIT ORGAN is formed out of a cavity in the soft tissues and bone of the face (*left*). A heat-sensitive membrane, 30 square millimeters in area but only 15 micrometers thick, is stretched across the cavity. The membrane intercepts infrared radiation that passes through the aperture of the pit. Inside the pit membrane (*right*) the bushy nerve endings of the trigeminal-nerve fibers terminate within a few micrometers of the membrane's outer surface. A change in the membrane temperature of only .003 degree Celsius is sufficient to raise the firing rate of the trigeminal-nerve fibers. The biophysical mechanism that accounts for the response to heat is not known.

of the pit receptor. Bullock found that in the absence of a stimulus individual axons carry an irregular low-frequency barrage of action potentials. When the pit is suddenly illuminated with moderately strong infrared radiation, the frequency of the firing of the action potentials increases dramatically. The firing rate rises within 100 milliseconds of the onset of the stimulus, remains high for a brief time and then slowly decays back to nearly the background level. When the illumination is turned off, the firing rate temporarily drops below the background level, then slowly recovers to its prestimulus rate.

Bullock and his colleagues found that individual axons are remarkably sensitive to infrared stimuli. A small warm object such as a human hand or a live rat, introduced as far as half a meter from the pit, triggers a noticeable increase in the firing rate of some of the trigeminal-nerve fibers. Such a stimulus corresponds to an increase of the energy incident on the pit organ of approximately .1 milliwatt per square centimeter. For the purpose of comparison, on a clear winter day in the northern U.S. the sun's rays deliver about 50 milliwatts of infrared per square centimeter.

Bullock and F. P. J. Diecke also made direct measurements of the temperature sensitivity of the trigeminal fiber endings in the rattlesnake pit organ. They controlled the internal temperature of the pit by directing a stream of warm water into the pit cavity. A change in the temperature of the flowing water as small as .003 degree Celsius produced a noticeable change in the firing rate of the more sensitive nerve fibers!

The pit organ's remarkable sensitivity to radiant heat can be traced to its remarkable structure. Each pit organ of a rattlesnake or boid snake consists of a cavity from one millimeter to five millimeters in diameter in the soft tissue and bone of the head. In rattlesnakes a thin membrane about 30 square millimeters in area is suspended across the air-filled space of the cavity. Only 15 micrometers thick, or about a fourth the thickness of this page, the membrane is the key component of the sense organ. Distributed across the membrane surface are some 7,000 thermosensitive endings of trigeminal sensory axons. Each of the endings can excite its nerve fiber if it is warmed. Similar heat-sensitive nerve endings cover the bottom of each pit in boid snakes. In boids the sensitive epithelium is not suspended in air as it is in rattlesnakes. The axon endings, however, come to within 30 micrometers of the surface.

The extreme heat sensitivity of the pit organs is a direct result of the proximity of the thermoreceptors to the outward-facing surface of the sensory epithelium. Infrared radiation falling on the surface immediately raises the tempera-

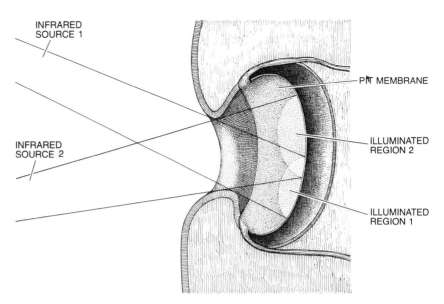

OPTICS OF THE PIT ORGAN resemble a pinhole camera. The diameter of the pit opening in a rattlesnake is about two millimeters, or roughly a third the diameter of the heat-sensitive membrane. Hence the radiation from an infrared source will illuminate only the area of membrane that falls within a cone defined by the location of the source and the pit aperture. Accuracy of the system is limited only by the snake's ability to localize edges of illuminated region.

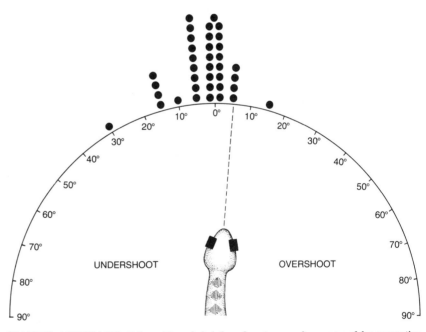

SPATIAL ACCURACY of the rattlesnake's infrared system can be measured by presenting a warm object at various angles to the left or the right of a snake whose eyes are covered with blinders. Each filled circle represents a single strike of the snake and shows the angular error between the strike and the target. The stimuli were presented at up to 60 degrees to the left or the right of the animal. The average error of the strikes is less than five angular degrees.

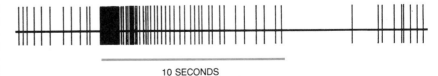

10 SECONDS

TRIGEMINAL-NERVE FIBERS signal changes in the temperature of the rattlesnake's pit membrane. The colored bar indicates a 10-second test period during which a snake's pit organ was exposed to infrared radiation. The traces on the line above the bar show the impulses recorded from a single trigeminal-nerve fiber. The firing rate is highest when the radiation is turned on but drops to nearly the background level. When the radiation is turned off, there is a short silent period. The properties of infrared trigeminal-nerve fibers were originally discovered by Theodore H. Bullock and his colleagues at the University of California at Los Angeles.

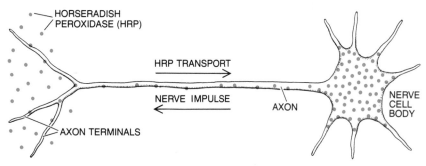

ANATOMICAL PATHWAY OF THE INFRARED SYSTEM was traced with the aid of an enzyme extracted from horseradish, horseradish peroxidase (HRP), which is taken up by the terminals of neurons and transported back to their cell bodies. HRP molecules are colored dots.

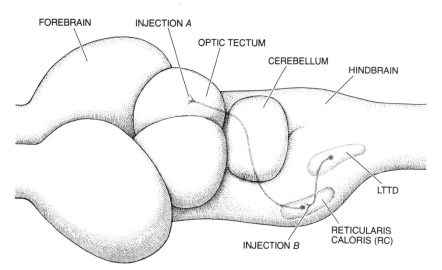

HORSERADISH PEROXIDASE INJECTED INTO BRAIN of a rattlesnake was traced by staining thin slices of tissue to reveal the presence of the enzyme. HRP injected into the optic tectum (*A*) was transported to a previously unknown nucleus, or collection of cell bodies, called the nucleus reticularis caloris (RC). When HRP was injected into the RC nucleus (*B*), stained cell bodies were found in the LTTD nucleus, which was known to receive a direct input from the pit organ. LTTD stands for a Latin expression that translates as "nucleus of the lateral descending trigeminal tract." The HRP experiments solved the puzzle of how the infrared information originating in the rattlesnake's pit organ ultimately reaches the optic tectum.

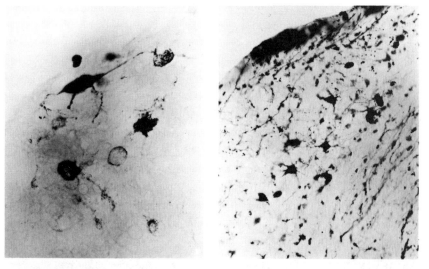

MICROGRAPHS OF BRAIN SLICES show how cell bodies labeled with HRP stand out as dark, irregular profiles after staining. The micrograph at the left is a section of the RC nucleus after horseradish peroxidase was injected into the optic tectum. The micrograph at the right is a section of the LTTD nucleus after the enzyme was injected into the RC nucleus. The experiments were done by the authors and Edward R. Gruberg of the Massachusetts Institute of Technology. Earl Kicliter of the University of Puerto Rico collaborated on first experiment.

ture of the sensors. The same amount of radiation falling on the bare skin of a mammal would raise the temperature of the first few micrometers of the skin by about the same amount. The thermoreceptors of mammals, however, lie much deeper. The entire thickness of the tissue between the surface and the receptors, about 300 micrometers, must be heated in order to warm them, and it takes 20 times as much heat energy to warm a layer of tissue 300 micrometers thick as it does to warm a layer only 15 micrometers thick. The sensitivity of mammalian thermoreceptors is further reduced by conductive heat loss to even deeper layers. Rattlesnakes avoid this problem with yet another specialization: since the heat-sensing membrane is surrounded by air on both sides, it does not lose heat to deeper tissues. Energy absorbed from infrared radiation almost exclusively heats the receptors.

Although the temperature sensitivity of rattlesnake trigeminal-nerve axons is impressive, it is not extraordinary when it is compared with the thermosensitive nerve cells of other animals. The skin of the human forehead, for example, has about the same threshold sensitivity to temperature. The great difference between rattlesnakes and other animals in sensitivity to incident radiation is primarily due to the anatomical specializations of the sensory organ and not to physiological differences in the sensory receptors.

The directional capabilities of the infrared sense can also be attributed to anatomical specializations of the pit. The pit organs of rattlesnakes have openings that are less than half the diameter of the sensory surface. Thus a small warm object half a meter or so in front of the pit will illuminate no more than a fourth of the entire thermosensitive membrane. The location of the illuminated patch on the membrane surface should therefore give an adequate clue to the location of a warm object. In short, the pit organ functions much like a crude pinhole camera.

The accuracy with which the snake can localize a warm object must depend on how accurately it can determine the position of the illuminated patch on the membrane. Simple trigonometric calculations show that in order to localize a small source to within five degrees of angle the snake must be able to measure the position of the warm spot on its receptive membrane to within about 175 micrometers. With a mosaic of receptors, each one about 60 micrometers across, such accuracy is quite reasonable. Diffraction of the infrared radiation (whose dominant wavelengths are in the band between six and 12 micrometers) may blur the edges of the warm spot somewhat, but not enough to reduce the pit's accuracy significantly.

Specializations evolved by the infrared-sensitive snakes are not limited to the pit organ. Pit vipers and boid snakes have also developed unique brain structures to process the novel information gathered by the pits. Early neurophysiological experiments on the rattlesnake brain demonstrated that the activity of many neurons (nerve cells) in the optic tectum of the midbrain (which was then thought to be primarily concerned with vision) was controlled by infrared stimuli. Evidently the infrared system, in parallel with its evolution from a facial-skin sense to a visionlike remote sense, has achieved a prominent representation in the tectum. This discovery, made independently by one of us (Hartline), who was then working at the University of California at San Diego, and by S.-I. Terashima and R. C. Goris of the Tokyo Medical and Dental University, presented an interesting anatomical problem. In other reptiles and in mammals the trigeminal nerve terminates in the trigeminal region of the hindbrain. How does infrared information originating in the trigeminal nerve find its way to the optic tectum of the midbrain in the rattlesnake?

Two groups of investigators began to work on the problem. Dolores M. Schroeder and Loop, working at the University of Virginia Medical School, employed cobalt ions to trace the connections of the rattlesnake trigeminal nerve. They placed the cut end of a branch of the nerve serving the pit in a cobalt chloride solution and passed an electric current between the solution and the brain. The current drove cobalt ions up the axons of the nerve to the axon terminals. When Schroeder and Loop treated sections of brain with a cobalt stain, they found that the trigeminal-nerve fibers, instead of ending in the normal trigeminal hindbrain area, ended in a new nucleus, now known as the LTTD (an abbreviation for the new structure, originally named in Latin "nucleus of the lateral descending trigeminal tract").

G. J. Molenaar of the University of Leiden independently identified what is almost certainly the same nucleus in the python, a boid snake. The LTTD nucleus appears to be peculiar to snakes that have a specialized infrared capability; it has been found in no other animal. It seems to be exclusively devoted to the infrared sensory system.

Our curiosity was piqued. If the nerve impulses carried by the trigeminal axons are delivered to the LTTD nucleus, what is the pathway that relays the infrared sensory information to the optic tectum? One approach to tracing connections within the brain is to use the peroxidase enzyme extracted from horseradish. The large horseradish-peroxidase molecule is taken up specifically by the axon terminals of individual neurons and is transported to other parts

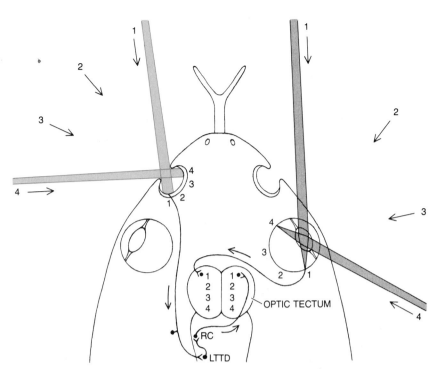

INFRARED SPACE AND VISUAL SPACE are represented in similar orientations on the surface of a rattlesnake's optic tectum. For clarity the pathways of the two sensory systems are depicted for opposite sides of the head. The front area of the tectum (1) receives input from the back areas of the pit membrane and from the retina, which survey roughly the same regions of space. The back area of the optic tectum (4) receives input from the front areas of the pit and the retina, which both "look" toward the side and behind the animal. Although the representations of the infrared and visual fields of view on the surface of the optic tectum have some systematic differences, they are similar enough so that each region of the optic tectum receives information through both sensory modalities from the same general region of space.

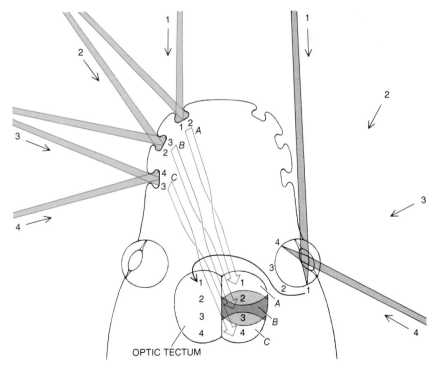

CONNECTIVITY IN THE PYTHON INFRARED SYSTEM is more complex than it is in the rattlesnake. The python pit organs look out on different but overlapping areas of infrared space. (Only three pits of the multipit array are shown.) The field of view of each pit is displayed over the pit's projection region on the tectal surface. Anterior pits (A) are represented in the front of the tectum, the more posterior pits (C) toward the rear of the tectum. The front area of each pit's infrared-sensitive epithelium is connected to the back of its projection region. The complex pattern of connections yields a more or less continuous representation of infrared space on the python's tectal surface that corresponds fairly well with the visual representation.

of the same cells. A staining procedure makes the horseradish peroxidase clearly visible in slices of brain and reveals the locations of the cell bodies of the neurons that took up the peroxidase.

Working with Edward R. Gruberg of the Massachusetts Institute of Technology and Earl Kicliter of the University of Puerto Rico, we injected horseradish peroxidase deep into the rattlesnake optic tectum where infrared sensory input is found. If cells in the LTTD projected directly to the optic tectum, we reasoned, their axon terminals in the tectum would pick up the peroxidase and transport it back to the LTTD. Somewhat to our surprise we found no stained neurons in the LTTD. Instead we found a group of prominently stained cells in a different region of the hindbrain. We postulated that this group of cells, which we named the nucleus reticularis caloris (RC), served as a relay station between the LTTD and the tectum.

Now we had to determine whether or not our new nucleus was connected directly to the LTTD. We investigated this question with Gruberg by injecting horseradish peroxidase into the RC nucleus. This time we did find stained cells in the LTTD. Stanford and Schroeder looked into the same question with a technique based on the degeneration of nerve cells. They selectively destroyed the cells of the rattlesnake LTTD nucleus and used a staining procedure that revealed the degenerated axons of these cells. They were able to trace the axons from the LTTD to the RC. Therefore both experimental approaches yielded the same answer: cells of the LTTD nucleus project directly to the RC. Although neither of these experiments could clarify the functional roles the LTTD nucleus and the RC nucleus play in the infrared sensory system, they at least explained how infrared information reaches the optic tectum. In the rattlesnake the LTTD and RC nuclei have evolved to process infrared sensory information and relay it to the tectum.

It is clear from the effectiveness of the infrared system in guiding the snake's strike that the system is able to localize objects in space with high accuracy. In this role it functions remarkably like the visual system of other animals. Our neurophysiological studies and those of our colleagues have revealed many similarities between the mechanisms that enable the visual and infrared systems to localize objects.

Bullock, and later J. A. DeSalvo, working with one of us (Hartline), described how individual trigeminal-nerve axons respond to warm stimuli anywhere within a field of view described by a cone originating at the pit. Such cones of view are usually between 45 and 60 degrees across and are called, by analogy with their visual counterparts in the retina, excitatory receptive fields. Most trigeminal fibers therefore behave as if their receptive fields were limited simply by the shadows cast by the lip of the pit. The response of any one trigeminal neuron would not convey the location of a stimulus accurately, but a population of many neurons, whose activity could be analyzed by the brain, might do so. In such analysis an important role is probably played by the optic tectum.

The optic tectum, also known in mammals as the superior colliculus, is one of the major visual centers of the brain. It is perhaps the main center for the processing of information about the location of objects in space. In monkeys the tectum helps to initiate and control "looking," or direction of gaze. In frogs and toads it probably initiates and controls the capture of flies and other prey.

In the optic tectum visual information is organized in an orderly way. Connections between the retina and the tectum (which are linked by the optic nerve) are made in such a way that a map of visual space is formed on the tectal surface. Just as a road map represents the spatial organization of roads on the earth's surface, so the visual map on the tectal surface represents space as it is viewed by the eye. For example, the front part of the tectum represents the part of visual space in front of the animal; the back part of the tectum represents the space toward the side and the rear. The orderly representation of visual space on the tectal surface is a constant feature of vertebrates, from fishes through primates.

Vision is not the only sense that can tell the brain where objects are. Sound also yields valuable location cues. So does touch. Both of these senses are also represented in the optic tectum of mammals. Furthermore, both the auditory system and the somatic sensory system are represented in the tectum in an orderly spatial way that coincides roughly with the visual system's tectal map. The front part of the tectum represents the front region of auditory space; sounds coming from in front of an animal preferentially excite this tectal region. Similarly, the front part of the tectum responds preferentially to touch stimulation of the front part of an animal such as the snout.

Is the infrared system organized in a similar spatial manner in the rattlesnake optic tectum? Leonard J. Kass, Loop and one of us (Hartline) investigated this question at the University of Illinois with the aid of neurophysiological techniques. We recorded the electrical responses of tectal cells from a grid

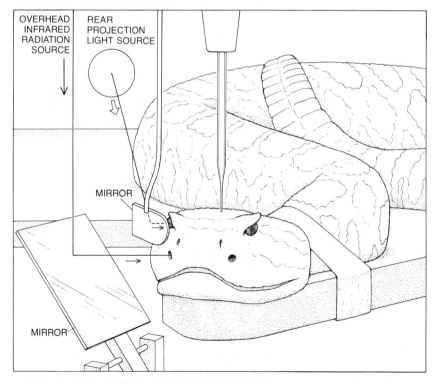

OVERHEAD INFRARED RADIATION SOURCE

REAR PROJECTION LIGHT SOURCE

MIRROR

MIRROR

RATTLESNAKE'S INFRARED AND VISUAL SENSES were stimulated with special equipment in the authors' laboratory at the Eye Research Institute of the Retina Foundation in Boston, Mass. The microelectrode above the snake's head recorded the activity of single tectal cells. Infrared radiation from a source directly above the snake was reflected off the large tiltable mirror and into the right pit organ. Visual images from a rear-projection screen were directed into the right eye by a smaller mirror. The visual stimulus was a bright circular spot.

of positions on the tectal surface and determined where in space an infrared stimulus elicited a maximal neuronal response.

After analyzing the data from several snakes we were gratified to discover not only that the infrared sense is organized spatially in the tectum but also that the infrared tectal map follows the same rules as the visual map. The front part of the tectum responds to infrared stimuli coming from in front of the snake; the back part, to stimuli coming from the side. In short, the visual and the infrared maps are, at least to a first approximation, in register. As we shall see, the similar spatial organizations of the visual and the infrared systems offer advantages in the processing of signals from the two sensory modalities.

The orientation of the map of infrared space on the tectum represents a major departure from the general vertebrate pattern of connections in the somatic sensory system, even though the infrared system presumably evolved from a somatic sense. In most other animals the front part of the tectum represents the front of the body surface. In the rattlesnake, however, the front part of the tectum represents the part of the pit membrane farthest from the animal's snout rather than the part nearest it. This inverted connectivity preserves in the tectum the normal representation of space but not of the body surface.

Boid snakes present an even more complex example of connectivity between the skin and the tectum. The reticulated python, for example, has 13 pits on each side of its head. Each pit is in essence an inverting optical system, which calls for an inverted tectal map, like the map in the rattlesnake. The pits toward the front of the python's head look farther forward, however, than the pits farther back along its lip. One would expect the front pits to be connected to the front part of the tectum, conforming to the usual noninverting vertebrate scheme. How, then, can the array of pits be connected to the tectum to form a reasonable representation of infrared space there? E. C. Haseltine of Indiana University tackled this intriguing problem in collaboration with one of us (Hartline).

What we found is the most complex somatic connectivity scheme observed in any animal to date. First we located the region of the tectum that receives connections from the entire sensory surface of a single pit, that is, the pit's projection region. When we mapped the pit's connections within that region, we found that the back part of each pit's sensory surface mapped to the front of its projection region in the tectum. The map of each pit is therefore inverted compared with the somatic maps of typical vertebrates. When we compared the projection regions of the different pits,

however, we found that the usual vertebrate mapping scheme holds true: the front pits project to the front of the tectum and the back pits project to the back. There is a final bit of complexity: adjacent pits, whose fields of infrared view overlap substantially, have substantially overlapping projection regions in the tectum.

The end result is a single, coherent representation of infrared space on the python tectal surface. Most important, the visual and the infrared maps in the python tectum correspond fairly well to each other. Evidently an intricate rearrangement of the connections between the somatic sensory system and the tectum has evolved to preserve the spatial registration between the two sensory modalities.

An intriguing possibility is suggested by the correspondence between the visual and the infrared representations of the world in the rattlesnake and python optic tectum. Perhaps the tectum compares or combines signals from the two senses. We knew that some tectal neurons in mammals are responsive to both visual and auditory stimuli or to both visual and tactile stimuli. We conjectured that similar "multimodal" neurons may exist in the rattlesnake tectum.

We were not disappointed. The first bimodal neurons in the tectum of a snake were identified by one of us (Hartline), Kass and Loop. The infrared stimuli were supplied by a hand or a warm soldering iron, the visual stimuli by a cardboard bar (which was thermally neutral). We found that some tectal neurons respond to warm objects whether the room is lighted or totally dark. The

same neurons respond to a cardboard bar, but only if the room lights are on. We called these cells "or" neurons, since they can be excited by stimulation of either of the two modalities.

We also found a small number of tectal neurons that respond to warm objects, but only if the room is lighted. These neurons do not respond to a thermally neutral cardboard bar even when the room is brightly lighted. Nor do they respond to a warm object in a darkened room. They were designated "and" neurons, since both visual and infrared stimuli seem to be essential for their response. Neurons such as these had never been described for any combination of sensory modalities in other animals.

The two of us (Newman and Hartline) realized that we might find other kinds of interactions of the visual and the infrared modalities if we tested specifically for them. We built a computer-controlled stimulator that could present infrared and visual stimuli whose intensity, location and time courses were independent of one another. Like some illusions of magic, this one was achieved with a few well-placed mirrors [*see illustration on page 20*].

In a typical experiment we lowered a recording microelectrode into the optic tectum of a rattlesnake and advanced it until we could record the electrical responses of a single neuron. Our computer then generated a sequence of infrared, visual and combined infrared-visual stimuli and recorded the responses from the cell. We then advanced the microelectrode until another cell was encountered. In this way we sampled and tested several scores of neurons.

Our hunch about possible exotic mo-

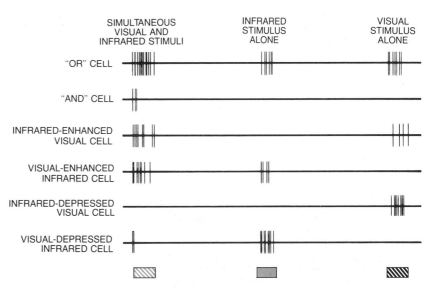

SIX CLASSES OF TECTAL CELLS that respond to infrared and visual stimuli have been identified. The rectangles on the bottom line show the time courses of combined infrared and visual stimuli (*color with white hatching*), infrared stimuli alone (*color*) and visual stimuli alone (*white hatching on black*). Tectal cells classed as "or," "and" and "enhanced" exhibit excitatory interactions of infrared and visual inputs. Two "depressed" classes of cells respond to only one of the two stimuli and show inhibitory interactions when both inputs are presented together.

dality interactions turned out to be well-founded. We discovered a number of novel infrared-visual interactions. The responses of the tectal cells, and therefore the cells themselves, fall naturally into six classes, two of which are represented by the "or" and "and" neurons. We confirmed that "or" cells respond to both infrared and visual stimuli presented alone as well as to combined infrared-visual stimuli. "And" cells respond only to simultaneous infrared-visual stimulation.

Tectal neurons of two other classes exhibit "enhancing" interactions of visual and infrared modalities. We describe such cells as "visual-enhanced infrared" cells or as "infrared-enhanced visual" cells, depending on the stimulus that does the enhancing. For example, a "visual-enhanced infrared" cell will show a moderate response (say four nerve impulses) to an infrared stimulus presented alone and will show no response to a visual stimulus. When infrared and visual stimuli are presented together, however, a larger response (eight impulses) is evoked. The excitatory influence of the visual stimulus, although the stimulus is not strong enough to generate a response by itself, can significantly enhance the cell's response to the infrared stimulus. Similarly, an "infrared-enhanced visual" cell will show no

response to an infrared stimulus but will show an enhanced response to a visual stimulus when it is accompanied by an infrared stimulus.

Tectal neurons of the remaining two classes display inhibitory interactions of the infrared and the visual modalities. The neurons of one class, which we call "infrared-depressed visual" cells, respond vigorously to a visual stimulus presented alone but fail to respond or responded weakly to the combined infrared-visual stimulus. The inhibitory influence of the infrared stimulus reduces or completely suppresses the response to the visual one. On the other hand, with cells of this class the removal of a warm object or the introduction of a cold one will enhance visual responses. The neurons of the other class, in which an infrared response is inhibited by a visual stimulus, we call "visual-depressed infrared" cells.

What functional role might be played by the infrared-visual neurons we have identified? Let us try to answer the question by considering how the tectum might function when a rattlesnake is searching out its prey. A simplified description of such behavior might divide it into several processes: the detection and localization of a stimulus, the identification of the stimulus and the triggering of the appropriate orientation move-

ment. An "attentional" process may also be involved in which the animal's attention is focused preferentially on one region of space; a stimulus in that region would trigger a movement of the head or the eyes but an equivalent stimulus in another region would not.

"Or" cells and "enhanced" cells would be useful in the detection process. "Or" cells would signal events in a particular region of space regardless of whether the events are perceived by way of the visual or infrared modalities or by way of both modalities at once. "Or" and enhanced cells respond more strongly to combined stimulation than to stimulation evoked by either visible or infrared radiation alone. Detection and localization would be improved by such excitatory interactions, particularly when neither modality is strongly excited. This might be the case if in the dim light of dusk a mouse was near the maximum detectable distance for the pit organ. Modality summation would occur at the correct tectal location because of the similar spatial organizations of the infrared and the visual modalities.

"Or" neurons and "enhanced" neurons might also be involved in an attentional process, one in which a warm, visible object to one side of a snake might catch the "attention" of the orientation machinery of the brain. The infrared

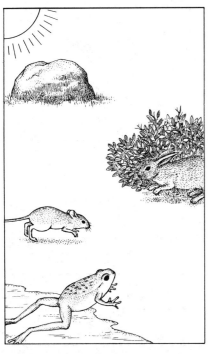

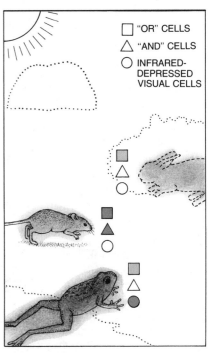

HYPOTHETICAL WORLD VIEWS perceived by a rattlesnake are represented schematically. The picture at the left depicts a scene as it might be recorded by the snake's visual system. The picture in the middle is the same scene as it might be perceived through the snake's infrared system. Only objects that are warm (*color*) or cool (*gray*) and moving would be detected. Stationary objects such as the bush and the pond would not be represented because they do not stimulate the infrared system well. Even the sun-warmed rock would be absent from the infrared image because it is also stationary. The images would be blurred because of the poor imaging properties of the pit organ. The

picture at the right suggests how the optic tectum might analyze the combined input of the two sensory systems. Responses of three of the six classes of bimodal tectal cells are represented by squares, triangles and circles. "Or" cells would be strongly activated (*solid color*) by the warm, clearly visible mouse and activated less intensely (*light color*) by the infrared component of the rabbit, which is hard to see against the bush, and by the visual component of the cool frog. "And" cells would be activated only by the mouse, which is both warm and clearly visible. The frog's cool skin would serve to disinhibit the "infrared-depressed visual" cells and cause them to respond strongly.

component of the stimulus would generate an elevated excitatory state among "or" and enhanced units in a large tectal region because infrared receptive fields are fairly large. Such a heightened excitation could prime that region of the tectum for visual stimulation by the same object or a nearby one. The infrared stimulation would thereby serve to draw attention to the corresponding part of visual space.

Infrared-visual tectal interactions might also contribute to the identification process by stimulating "feature-detecting" neurons that respond only to specific combinations of infrared and visual stimuli. "And" cells, for example, are activated only by objects that can be detected by the pit organ and simultaneously by the eye. Such simultaneous stimulation causes "and" neurons to give a brief but high-frequency burst of impulses. We have found that the most effective stimulus for these cells is a small, warm, moving object. These neurons might be described whimsically as mouse detectors.

Infrared-depressed visual cells, on the other hand, respond best to thermally neutral or cool visual objects: leaves fluttering in a breeze or perhaps a frog jumping at a pond's edge. The visual activity of these cells would be depressed by the infrared radiation of warm-blooded animals. In such examples cross-modality interactions are essential for correct identification of the stimulus.

The cross-modality interactions we have described show that in the rattlesnake tectum the infrared and visual sense modalities are integrated to a significant degree. Could similar modality-combining interactions be operating in the optic tectums of other species? Are tactile and auditory signals in mammals combined in complex ways with visual input? We simply do not know. The experiments necessary to identify such interactions have not been done. We would be willing to bet, however, that the kinds of modality interactions we have observed in snakes are present and functionally important in the tectums of most other vertebrates.

It is ironic that so little is known about how the infrared sense is exploited by snakes in their natural habitat. No one knows whether rattlesnakes and pythons make use of their infrared detectors to hunt prey during the day, when their visual system is also operational. Nor is it known whether snakes rely on their infrared system to identify predators and to locate a comfortable resting place. These are interesting questions for the future. For the present it is impressive enough to know that in the pit vipers and the boid snakes the trigeminal skin sense has evolved into a sensitive distance sense that is much like vision itself.

3

The Compound Eye
of Insects

by G. Adrian Horridge
July 1977

*It has hundreds of facets, each representing an ommatidium,
or "little eye." The size, pattern, and aiming of the ommatidia
are determined by the requirements of the insect's way of life*

Insects are legion; some are active only in bright sunlight, some in both sunlight and shade, some only at twilight. Some, such as the common housefly, travel at high speed and make rapid turns. Others, such as the dragonfly, alternately fly straight, maneuver and hover. Still others, such as the praying mantis, remain motionless for hours at a time. All these insects rely for their survival on vision, and all of them perceive the world through many-faceted compound eyes, yet their habits and their visual requirements are quite different. How does the compound eye work as an optical sampling device? To what extent does it reveal the functions for which the insect uses its eyes? To what extent does the smallness of the facets of the insect eye limit its sensitivity? What is the barrier to the insect eye's working at low light intensities with the small lenses of the facets? How do the compound eyes of insects arrive at a compromise between optical resolution and the sensitivity needed to overcome optical noise?

A compound eye is made up of ommatidia: tiny individual eyes that point in different directions. Each ommatidium consists of a lens that focuses light on several receptor cells sharing the common light-sensitive organ known as a rhabdom. In many insects each ommatidium is a single sampling element with its own optical axis; only insect eyes with this type of ommatidium will be discussed here. Light absorbed by the rhabdom transmits a signal to the insect's brain through an optic nerve. Another question is: How can we determine the directions in which the ommatidia are looking? And what does that tell us about how the insect perceives the world?

Looking at the eye of an insect, we frequently see a black spot in the center of the eye. As the insect rotates its head the black spot always points in the direction of the observer. The spot is known as the pseudopupil; the facets in it look black because they reflect less light in the direction of the observer than the facets in the rest of the eye do. In other words, the ommatidia in the center of the pseudopupil are looking directly at the observer.

To map the optical axis of each ommatidium the head of the insect (or the entire animal) is mounted at the center of a goniometer, a device for measuring angles. The angle required to move the center of the pseudopupil a distance of five facets is measured, and the measurement is repeated at intervals of five facets until the entire eye is mapped. The same data can be more easily collected by photographing the eye at intervals of five or 10 degrees. In that case the facets are marked with dust particles, and the positions of the pseudopupil with respect to the pattern of the marked facets are measured from the photographs. The position of the axis of each fifth facet is then plotted on a grid in angular coordinates. The resulting pattern is a map of the way in which the compound eye samples the visual world. So far only a few partial maps have been made, such as one prepared for the housefly by the Dutch biophysicists D. G. M. Beersma, Doekele G. Stavenga and Jan W. Kuiper. Only narrow strips can be mapped without encountering the familiar problems that are encountered in mapping a sphere on a flat piece of paper.

Two angles are of prime importance in understanding the function of an insect eye. The first is the angle between the optical axes of two adjacent ommatidia. This is the interommatidial angle, denoted $\Delta\phi$, which determines how densely the compound eye samples the visual world. The second is the angle defining the field of view of a single ommatidium, denoted $\Delta\rho$. The shape of the field is in effect the sensitivity of the ommatidium to a point source of light as a function of angle from the optical axis. The sensitivity of the ommatidium is at its greatest along the optical axis, and it decreases with angle from the axis. The width of the field is defined as the angle subtended by the diameter across the field where the sensitivity has dropped to 50 percent.

The eye maps reveal some surprises about the way in which insects perceive the world. First, the maps show that the pattern of the optical axes is not the same as the pattern of the hexagonal facets on the surface of the eye. Facets that are an equal distance apart on the surface of the eye do not necessarily have optical axes that are at the same interommatidial angle. In fact, in one region of the eye the optical axes of the ommatidia may be tilted toward one another so that they are nearly parallel, thus giving one segment of the visual world more than its share of the distribution of sampling points. In that region the pseudopupil is usually larger than it is elsewhere on the eye, because more facets are looking in that direction.

Such an area on the compound eye of insects has the same function as the fo-

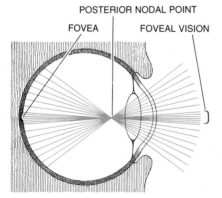

POSTERIOR NODAL POINT

FOVEA   FOVEAL VISION

EYE OF A VERTEBRATE ANIMAL has a small cup-shaped area in the retina where vision is particularly acute. In that area, the fovea centralis, the visual receptors are closely packed, so that their resolution, or ability to distinguish fine detail, is high. Each line in color represents the optical axis of every *n*th receptor. The close packing of the receptors in the fovea requires that the receptors be narrow, so that the sensitivity of each foveal receptor is lower than that of the receptors elsewhere in the retina. Hence the fovea in vertebrate animals is a specialized area for seeing with high resolution only in bright light.

vea centralis in the retina of vertebrate animals (including man). In vertebrates the fovea is an area where the visual receptors are packed closer together, providing the most acute vision. Indeed, in the eyes of diurnal animals (including man) the receptors must be very narrow to be so closely packed, and the sensitivity of each receptor is correspondingly reduced. Hence in vertebrates the fovea is an adaptation for acute vision in bright light.

In insects, however, the facets in the fovea are usually larger than those over the rest of the eye. Since the interommatidial angle in the fovea is reduced, the region of the eye that includes the fovea is optically flatter than the rest of the eye; in other words, it has a larger radius of curvature than the rest of the eye. Thus for there to be room for a fovea in one region of a compound eye the eye must have a smaller optical radius of curvature elsewhere. The result is that some areas of the eye are impoverished in sampling points so that another area can be enriched.

Larger facets make it possible for their ommatidia to have a higher resolving power. For any lens the capability to resolve fine detail depends on two factors: the aperture or diameter of the lens (D), and the wavelength (λ) of the light focused through it. (Because of the difficulty in measuring the aperture of a hexagonal lens, D is taken as the distance between centers of adjacent facets.) Light from a distant point source passing through the lens is not focused to a point but is blurred into a circle in the focal plane of the lens. The intensity of the light in this blur circle is greatest in

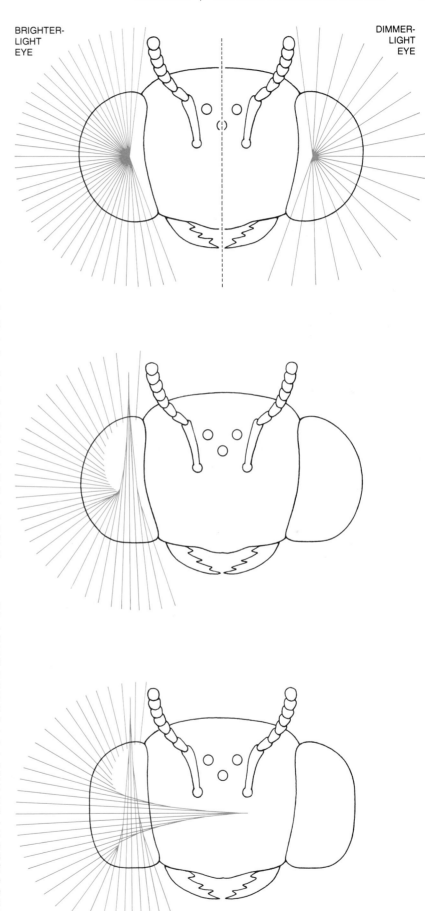

COMPOUND EYE OF AN INSECT is built up of ommatidia. The effective size of any part of such an eye is established by its optical radius, which is defined as the radius measured from the point where the optical axes of adjacent ommatidia intersect. Here four types of compound eye are seen from above the back of the insect. If the insect eye were a hemisphere and ommatidia of equal aperture looked out perpendicularly to the surface of the eye, the entire eye would have one optical radius, and it would sample the visual world with equal density in all directions (*top*). The sensitivity of a compound eye depends partly on the size of its facets and therefore on its overall size for a given number of facets. Measurements of actual compound eyes indicate, however, that in many of them the optical radius at the front of the eye is greater than it is elsewhere on the eye (*middle*). Therefore the part of the visual world seen by the front of the eye is sampled more densely than other parts are. Such an area is called a fovea by analogy with the fovea of the vertebrate eye. At the fovea of most insect eyes the facets are larger, which is made possible by the eye's having a greater optical radius. Some insects (*bottom*) have a second fovea that looks upward or to the side; large dragonflies have foveas of all three kinds.

the center and falls off toward the edge. It is convenient to define the width of the blur circle as the diameter where the intensity of the light has fallen to 50 percent. That width is denoted $\Delta\alpha$. From diffraction theory it is known that the angular width of the blur circle in radians is equal to the wavelength of the light divided by the diameter of the lens ($\Delta\alpha = \lambda/D$). (One radian is a full circle divided by π, or approximately 57 degrees.) Hence for any particular wavelength of light, the larger the lens, the smaller the blur circle for each point source and the sharper the image.

There is much evidence that in insects relying on acute vision the optical performance of the lens of each ommatidium is excellent, and that the receptor structure catching the light (which is in effect the tip of the rhabdom) lies in the focal plane of the lens. There are two fundamental limits on the resolution of the individual ommatidium. The first is the width of the blur circle: a large facet on an insect's eye can have a higher resolving power than a small one because it concentrates the light into a smaller blur circle. The second limit has to do with how narrow the receptor can be and still act as a light guide; the minimum diameter of the receptor is about .5 micrometer.

If a point source of light lies on the optical axis of the ommatidium, the most intense, or brightest, portion of the blur circle will be centered on the tip of the rhabdom. As the point source travels across the field of view, it moves away from the optical axis and the peak of the blur circle moves away from the rhabdom. Thus the rhabdom will intercept a progressively smaller and less intense segment of the blur circle. If the rhabdom is relatively narrow, it can precisely measure the variation in the intensity of the light across the blur circle, and its resolution is limited only by the diffraction of the light that gave rise to the blur circle.

By the same token, however, a narrow rhabdom will capture only a small fraction of the total light in the blur circle and its sensitivity will be low. If the rhabdom is wider, it will capture more of the light in the blur circle, but its resolution will be poorer because it will not be able to measure detail as well. Hence the optimum angular sensitivity of the rhabdom is a function both of the width $\Delta\alpha$ of the blur circle and the diameter d of the rhabdom. In every eye there is a compromise between resolution, which is limited only by the diffraction or the minimum rhabdom width, and sensitivity, which, as we shall see, is very important in eyes with such small lenses.

This compromise can be illustrated by an analogy: the way in which the profile of a spray of water from a shower head can be measured by containers of different sizes. The diameter of the spray is equivalent to the width of the blur circle, and the water drops are equivalent to the photons of light. A small bowl moved across the spray will readily measure, or resolve, the intensity profile of the spray, or will readily distinguish the boundaries of several sprays that are close together. Yet at any point the bowl will intercept only a small portion of the spray, that is, its sensitivity is low. The spray is caught much more effectively by a large tub. The tub is thus more "sensitive" than the bowl, yet by catching so much of the water it cannot distinguish detail or discriminate between sprays that are close together. When the flow is low, however, only large sprays can be detected, and the tub provides the best means for measuring the distribution of the spray.

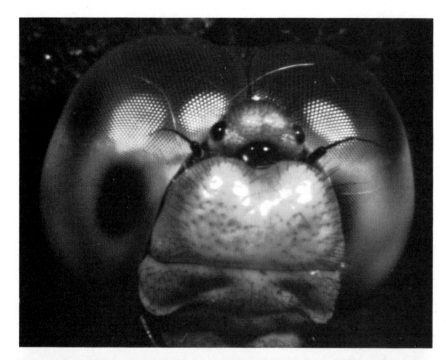

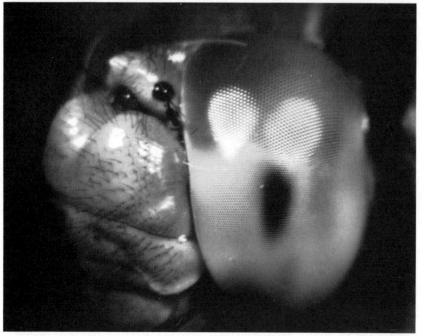

PSEUDOPUPIL OF INSECT EYE is seen as a black spot on the eye of the libellulid dragonfly *Diplacodes nematodes*. As the insect's head turns, the pseudopupil moves so that it always points toward the observer. The pseudopupil is black because the facets in that area reflect less light in the direction of the observer than the facets in other areas of the eye. The facets in the center of the pseudopupil are looking directly at the observer. In general, where the pseudopupil is larger (*top*) more ommatidia are looking in that direction. At the side of the eye (*bottom*) the pseudopupil is elongated vertically because the optical axes in vertical rows have between them about half the angle found between the visual axes of the ommatidia in horizontal rows.

If the diameter d of a circular rhabdom is narrow compared with the width of the blur circle $\Delta\alpha$, the rhabdom's field of view $\Delta\rho$ is equal to the angular width of the blur circle. If the rhabdom is wide enough to catch 95 percent of all the light in the blur circle, the rhabdom's field of view $\Delta\rho$ turns out to be twice the angular width of the blur circle at 50 percent intensity, or $2\Delta\alpha$. Increasing the diameter of the rhabdom beyond that value results in a continuing loss in resolution without a corresponding increase in sensitivity to a point source of light. In the shower analogy, having a tub larger than the diameter of the spray will not increase the amount of water the tub can catch from one spray. Making the rhabdom "tub" larger, however, is obviously a better stratagem for seeing at least something when photons are so scarce that only large sprays of them can be detected.

So far in this discussion of the origin of the insect's field of view from the blur circle it has been necessary to avoid problems presented by the refraction, or bending, of light as it passes from the air into the insect's eye. Angles such as the width of the blur circle $\Delta\alpha$ (inside the eye) and the field of view (outside the eye) are measured from the posterior nodal point, which in a one-sided lens such as this one is a point very close to the center of curvature of the lens. Rays of light passing through the posterior nodal point inside the eye are parallel to the same rays outside the eye; for that reason the posterior nodal point is a useful one for relating angles measured outside the eye to angles measured inside the eye. The diameter of a large receptor subtended at the posterior nodal point is the size of the field of view $\Delta\rho$.

Let us suppose that in a typical ommatidium of high resolving power the lens is 28.5 micrometers in aperture. If the wavelength is .5 micrometer (the wavelength of green light), the width of the blur circle $\Delta\alpha$ is then one degree. If in such an ommatidium the diameter of the rhabdom (subtended at the posterior nodal point) were equal to the width of the blur circle at 50 percent intensity $\Delta\alpha$, then from the formula $\Delta\rho^2 = \Delta\alpha^2 + (d/f)^2$ its field of view would be 1.4 degrees. This rhabdom could have a diameter of one micrometer and a focal length f (measured from the posterior nodal point to the tip of the rhabdom) of 57 micrometers. A rhabdom with a diameter of less than a micrometer is not very effective as a light guide, and such narrow rhabdoms are rarely found in insect eyes. A larger aperture of facet would generate a narrower blur circle, calling for a narrower rhabdom. Therefore if the performance of the ommatidium is limited by the diffraction of light, one would not expect to find insects with ommatidia that have facets more than about 30 micrometers across, because effective rhabdoms cannot be

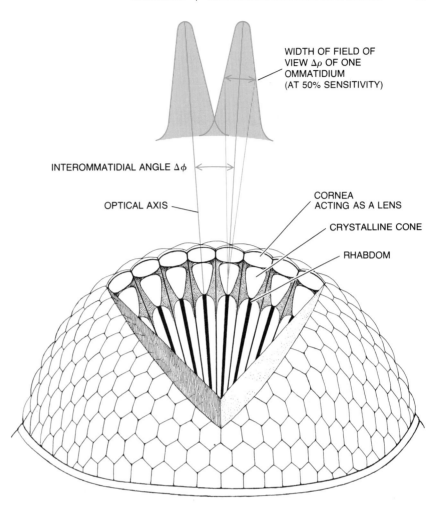

WIDTH OF FIELD OF VIEW $\Delta\rho$ OF ONE OMMATIDIUM (AT 50% SENSITIVITY)

INTEROMMATIDIAL ANGLE $\Delta\phi$

OPTICAL AXIS

CORNEA ACTING AS A LENS

CRYSTALLINE CONE

RHABDOM

STRUCTURE OF INSECT EYE determines how much detail the eye is capable of seeing. Each ommatidium has a cornea that also serves as a lens focusing light through a transparent cone onto a light-sensitive element: the rhabdom. The optical axis of the ommatidium is the line extending through the center of the lens to the rhabdom. The interommatidial angle $\Delta\phi$ is the angle between the optical axes of the adjacent ommatidia. The curves in color above each ommatidium indicate how the sensitivity of the ommatidium decreases with angular distance from the ommatidium's optical axis. The field of view of each of the ommatidia is defined as the angle subtended where the sensitivity has fallen to 50 percent of its maximum value.

made thin enough to match the facets.

The fact is, however, that facets up to 80 micrometers in diameter are commonly found, particularly in the fovea. Some organisms other than insects, such as the stomatopod mantid shrimp *Odontodactylus* and the deep-sea amphipod *Phronima*, have a compound eye with facets up to 120 micrometers across. All compound eyes have fewer and larger facets than the diffraction theory predicts. Why should such large apertures be found? The answer is that further increasing the diameter of the lens increases the ommatidium's sensitivity in proportion to the area of the lens (D^2). Consideration of point sources and the diffraction limit can take one no further in understanding the compound eye. The individual ommatidia seem to be adapted in many ways to catching every last photon of light. In the shower analogy one must turn from the process of catching a single small shower to distinguishing low-flow showers of all sizes in different combinations. When the flow

of drops (photons) is so low that only large showers can be detected, sensitivity is important.

So far I have concentrated on optical constraints and on the characteristics of a single ommatidium. A compound eye, however, is an array of hundreds of ommatidia looking out more or less equally in many directions. The advantage of such an arrangement is that it operates by parallel processing: it divides information from the external world into many parallel channels, analyzes the information in each channel and recombines some of the information in the brain. Thus an insect can be aware of its entire visual world at every moment, whereas vertebrate animals such as ourselves can gain that information only by continually moving their eyes and head in a series of scans.

What governs the spacing of the ommatidia over the surface of the eye? In 1894 A. Mallock (and later Horace B. Barlow, Hugo de Vries, Jan Kuiper and

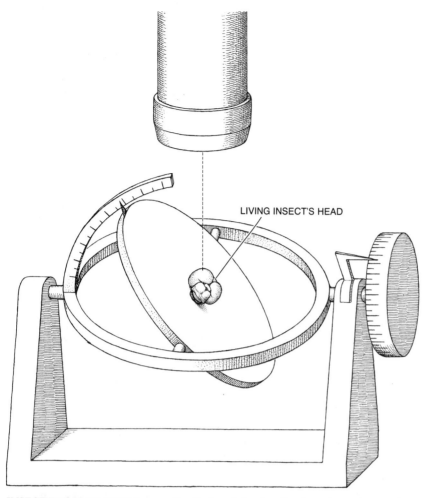

INSECT EYE IS MAPPED by mounting the insect's head on the stage of a goniometer (calibrated gimbals) and photographing the eye over a range of angles. The angle required to move the center of the pseudopupil five facets determines the interommatidial angle between every fifth ommatidium. Position of optical axes of each fifth ommatidium is then plotted on a map.

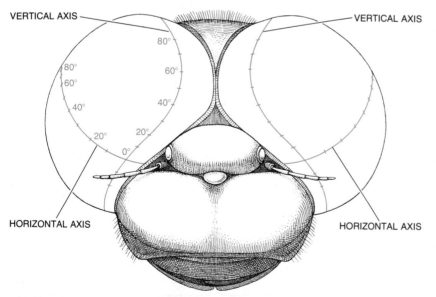

COORDINATE SYSTEM FOR MAPPING INSECT EYE is arbitrary, but the principal functional axes of the eye are used. The zero of the vertical axis usually crosses the zero of the horizontal axis at the position of the insect's forward-looking fovea. The zero vertical axis on the maps in angular coordinates is the line of facets that look in the plane in which the forward and vertical directions lie. It is not a straight line down the eye. The zero horizontal axis on the maps is the line joining the facets that look out horizontally. Again it is not necessarily a horizontal row of facets running across the eye because optical axes can be inclined to eye surface.

many others) proposed that the angular spacing of the ommatidia might be calculated from the limits of diffraction, in that the angular spacing of adjacent lenses ($\Delta\phi$) need be no better than twice the spacing ($\Delta\theta$) of the finest pattern each can resolve. The argument was basically the following:

The world the insect perceives can be regarded as a complex pattern of contrasts between light and dark. Such a pattern can be approximated as the sum of a number of regular patterns of stripes, each with a sinusoidal distribution of intensity between light and dark and a regular period $\Delta\theta$. For an array of receptors to see a striped pattern and reconstruct it as stripes by simultaneous parallel processing, the minimum angular spacing between receptors (that is, the interommatidial angle $\Delta\phi$) must be equal to the angle subtended by half the spacing of the striped pattern (that is, $\frac{1}{2}\Delta\theta$). With that minimum spacing two peaks (bright stripes) in the pattern of the stripes' intensity, together with the trough between them (a dark stripe), fall on three adjacent receptors. If the interommatidial angle were smaller, there would be more than enough receptors to discern the pattern; if the interommatidial angle were larger, there would be too few receptors to discern it. This idea is known as the Whittaker-Shannon sampling theorem, and in two dimensions it applies to receptors arrayed in a square pattern. As has been shown recently by Allan Snyder of the Australian National University and William H. Miller of the Yale University School of Medicine, for a hexagonal pattern of receptors to attain the same visual acuity as a square pattern, the hexagonal pattern needs more receptors by a factor of 2 divided by the square root of 3. The eye maps of insects reveal that the pattern of the optical axes of the ommatidia lies between the square and the hexagonal pattern. The hexagonal pattern is warped into a pattern of oblique squares, particularly around the equator of the eye.

From diffraction theory it is also known that the spacing of the stripes $\Delta\theta$ in the finest pattern that can be resolved at any wavelength of light through a lens of aperture D is equal to the wavelength of light λ divided by the aperture of the lens ($\Delta\theta = \lambda/D$). Since the minimum interommatidial angle $\Delta\phi$ must be equal to half the spacing of the stripes, then in order for a diffraction-limited eye to see, the product of the aperture of the lens and the interommatidial angle must be equal to half the wavelength of light (that is, $D\Delta\phi = \lambda/2$). The early workers thought that this was the case.

If we say, however, that the eye must operate at a higher level of light modulation to overcome photon noise, then we can say that $D\Delta\phi$ is equal to λ, so that $D\Delta\phi$ is now equal to .5 micrometer. The product $D\Delta\phi$ should therefore be constant for an eye that functions at a given modulation level, and it should be .25 micrometer for square patterns of axes working at the diffraction limit. Both D and $\Delta\phi$ can be measured from outside the eye. On the basis of simple geometry the interommatidial angle in radians is the facet diameter D divided by the optical radius R. Therefore D^2/R should be constant for eyes of different sizes that work at the same intensity. In other words, simply by knowing the aperture of the ommatidium's lens D and the interommatidial angle $\Delta\phi$ one can determine a great deal about the structure of the eye from the product of the two. That applies both for different insects and for different regions on the eye of a single insect.

If the structure of the compound eye of an insect were designed to reconstruct detail at the diffraction limit at a wavelength of .5 micrometer, then the eye parameter $D\Delta\phi$ would be fixed at a value of between .25 and .31, depending on how the pattern of the optical axes is distributed between squares and hexagons. The eye maps reveal, however, that there are no insects with compound eyes the structure of which is determined by these limits. Evidently sunlight is never bright enough to eliminate photon noise as a factor. Only the foveas of some insects that are active in bright sunlight approach the diffraction limit.

When a pattern of stripes with a spacing of $\Delta\theta$ passes across an insect's field of view, the rhabdom perceives the pattern as a modulation, or oscillation, laid over a mean intensity of light. If the spacing of the striped pattern $\Delta\theta$ is large in relation to the field width $\Delta\rho$, then the amplitude of the modulation from light to dark will also be large. If the spacing of the striped pattern is small, then the amplitude of the modulation will be small. The speed of movement is not important until levels are reached where the receptor fails to respond in time.

The mean light intensity depends on the ambient illumination of the stripes and the width of the field. The amplitude of the modulation M experienced by the receptor is in fact the amount by which the intensity of the light fluctuates from the mean intensity. Specifically, the relative modulation experienced by the receptor is equal to the difference of the maximum intensity and the minimum intensity divided by the sum of the maximum intensity and the minimum intensity. Thus a spatial modulation m in the contrast between light and dark in the visual world is converted by the motion and the receptor into a temporal modulation M, the relative amplitude of which depends on the width of the field of view, the spacing of the stripes and (at significant speeds) the angular velocity of the relative movement [see illustration on page 31].

A receptor with a broad field of view

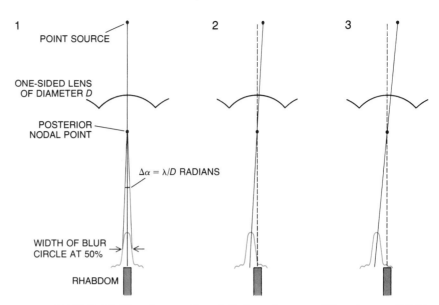

LIGHT IS DIFFRACTED as it passes through the lens of an ommatidium. As a result light from a point source is not focused to a point but forms a circular pattern, the blur circle. The intensity of the blur circle (*curves in color*) is greater in the center and falls off toward the edges. The width of the blur circle ($\Delta\alpha$) is defined as its diameter where the intensity has fallen to 50 percent. That angular width (in radians) is equal to the wavelength of light from a point source divided by the diameter D of the lens. When blur circle is on optical axis (*1*), rhabdom receives greatest amount of light. As point source moves away from optical axis (*2 and 3*), blur circle moves away from tip of the rhabdom and amount of light rhabdom receives decreases. The rays are drawn through the posterior nodal point, which is near center of curvature of lens. Rays passing through this point have a path inside eye that is parallel to their path outside it.

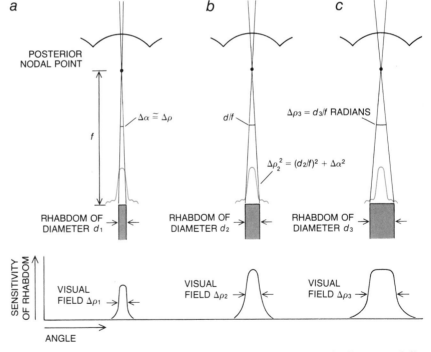

RHABDOM'S SENSITIVITY AND RESOLUTION are a function of its diameter and distance from the posterior nodal point. A narrow rhabdom (*a*) with a diameter d_1 less than the width of the blur circle at 50 percent intensity will receive only a fraction of the light in the blur circle, but it will respond well to the variation of light across the blur circle and thus will have high resolution but low sensitivity. An ommatidium with such a rhabdom is said to be near the diffraction limit. A wider rhabdom (*b*) with a diameter d_2 equal to twice the width of the blur circle will capture 95 percent of the light in the blur circle, but it will have a slightly wider field and therefore poorer resolution. An ommatidium (*c*) with a larger rhabdom diameter d_3 has a wide field of view that is no better than *b* for point sources, but it is better for detecting extended objects in dim light. The angular sensitivity, or shape of the field, of each rhabdom (measured across the width at 50 percent sensitivity) is shown in the curves at the bottom of the illustration. The sensitivity for large objects increases with rhabdom size in proportion to $(d/f)^2$ in the same way that photographic film is more sensitive when its grains are larger.

Δρ will catch more light and will have a better signal-to-noise ratio than a receptor with a narrow field of view (by a factor of Δρ²), but a receptor with a large field of view will also be less sensitive to the modulation produced by narrow stripes. Similarly, an ommatidium with a large facet diameter D will expe-

rience more absolute modulation by a factor D^2. An efficient transfer of the modulation into the eye is essential, particularly when the intensity of the ambient light is low. Therefore if one could determine the level of the light signal required to activate the receptors above the level of the light noise, one could

arrive at the optimum relation between the diameter of the facets and the interommatidial angle for insects that are active in different levels of light.

An extended light source of constant brightness is emitting an average number $\overline{N}$ of photons per unit of time. The photons nonetheless arrive at the rhabdom randomly; at any one moment the rhabdom may receive more than the average number of photons and at the next moment it may receive fewer than the average number. The variation in the actual number of photons from the average number of photons is the unavoidable noise; it is defined as the standard deviation from the average number of photons, and for light it is equal to the square root of the average number of photons, or $\sqrt{\overline{N}}$.

The absolute signal that the rhabdom actually receives is the relative amplitude of the modulation M multiplied by the average number of photons caught $M\overline{N}$. The ratio of the signal to the noise is therefore $M\overline{N}/\sqrt{\overline{N}}$, which is equal to $M\sqrt{\overline{N}}$. This ratio of the signal to the noise must be large enough for the signal to stand out above the noise, so that the ommatidium does not respond to false alarms. If $\overline{N}$ therefore decreases at the limit, M must correspondingly rise. If the rhabdom is receiving an average of, say, four photons per unit of time from a light source, the noise in that number of photons is plus or minus two photons; thus the modulation M in the average number of photons (the signal) must be greater than 50 percent of the average number of photons for the modulation to stand out above the noise. In bright light, however, the modulation can be lower as long as the product of $M\sqrt{\overline{N}}$ is still about 1. If the rhabdom is receiving an average of, say, 100 photons per unit of time, the noise is plus or minus 10 photons, so that the modulation M in the average number of photons need be only about 10 percent.

There are now enough equations to calculate the eye parameter $D\Delta\phi$ for any value of the ambient intensity of light, and the results appear as the smooth curve in the illustration on page 33 (which is from the recent work of Allan Snyder, Doekele Stavenga and Simon Laughlin). From that curve the amount by which the circles in the eye maps should overlap for optimum vision can be calculated for any intensity of ambient light. For a diffraction-limited eye, which must have an eye parameter of .3 or less, the circles of diameter λ/D on the eye maps must overlap each other almost halfway, and the actual field width $\Delta\rho$ should be twice the interommatidial angle $\Delta\phi$. For the eyes of insects that have an eye parameter of .5 the width of the field should be about 1.3 times larger than the interommatidial angle; for those with an eye parameter of 2 the width of the field $\Delta\rho$

EYE MAP shows the front part of the right eye of the gomphid dragonfly *Austrogomphus*, which has one fovea looking obliquely upward and forward. Each circle represents the narrowest possible field of each fifth ommatidium. To compensate for the factor of five the diameter is equal to five times the wavelength of green light (taken to be .5 micrometer) divided by the diameter of the ommatidium's lens, or $5\lambda/D$. Smaller circles mean that the facets in that area of the insect's eye are larger and have a higher resolution than those in areas with larger circles. The center of each circle represents the position of the optical axis of each fifth ommatidium; the distance from the center of one circle to the center of the next is hence equal to five times the interommatidial angle, or $5\Delta\phi$. Amount by which the circles are separated or overlap yields the value of the eye parameter $D\Delta\phi$, which is a critical measure of how far from the diffraction limit the insect's eye is in each area. In this eye there are only about a fourth of the number of facets there would be at the diffraction limit. Center of fovea is at the center of grouping of small circles near 0 degrees, 50 degrees on axes in angular space.

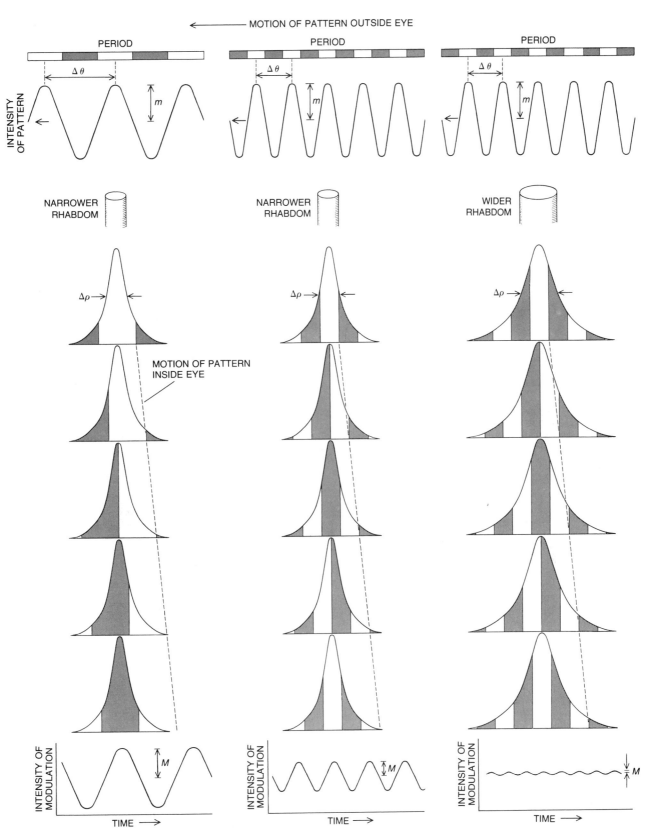

PATTERN OF DARK AND LIGHT STRIPES (*top*) moving across an ommatidium's field of view is perceived by the rhabdom as a modulation of the intensity of light in time. The stripes have a sinusoidal distribution of intensity of amplitude *m* from light to dark (*curves second from top*). The amount of modulation perceived by the rhabdom (*cylindrical structures third from top*) is a function of the rhabdom's field of view $\Delta\rho$ and of the stripes' spacing $\Delta\theta$. At the left a narrow rhabdom looks at a moving pattern of wide stripes; the rhabdom's field of view is a quarter of the period of the stripes ($\Delta\rho = \frac{1}{4}\Delta\theta$). The sensitivity of the rhabdom across its field of view is represented by the shape of the peaked curves below the cylindrical rhabdom structures. As the wide stripes move across the rhabdom's narrow field of view the rhabdom perceives a modulation of large amplitude *M* (*curve at bottom left*). In the middle a narrow rhabdom looks at a moving pattern of narrow stripes ($\Delta\rho = \frac{1}{2}\Delta\theta$) and perceives a faster modulation of moderate amplitude. At the right a wide rhabdom looks at a moving pattern of narrow stripes ($\Delta\rho = \Delta\theta$) and sees a rapidly flickering gray blur that could be below optical noise level for all conditions except the brightest illumination or the largest eye facets. The diagonal broken lines show the motion inside the eye.

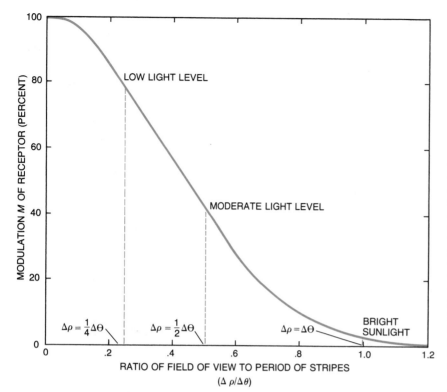

AMPLITUDE OF RELATIVE MODULATION M **perceived by the rhabdom as a striped pattern moves through its field of view is shown as a function of the ratio of the width of the field of view to the spacing of the stripes. When the field is equal to the spacing of the stripes ($\Delta\rho = \Delta\theta$), the modulation is only a few percent, which may be sufficient for vision in bright sunlight. When the field is equal to half the spacing ($\Delta\rho = \frac{1}{2}\Delta\theta$), modulation is about 40 percent, as would be required at lower light levels to overcome photon noise. Hence receptors for working at low light levels have large field ($\Delta\rho$), for which they must have large diameter (d).**

should be only three-quarters of the interommatidial angle $\Delta\phi$. Whether these field sizes are actually found in insect eyes must still be checked in a wide range of different kinds of insects.

The sensitivity of the insect eye can be increased by a factor D^2 by increasing the aperture D of the lens in the ommatidium or by a factor $(d/f)^2$ by decreasing the distance f from the posterior nodal point to the rhabdom. In either case the field of view is widened. In the compound eyes of large dragonflies, locusts, mantids, wasps and beetles (and also in the eyes of many crustaceans) the curvature of the lens is on the inside, so that the posterior nodal point is a little closer to the rhabdom and the eye can function equally well whether they are in water or out of it. The outside surface of the eye is then almost glassy smooth. In many insect eyes there is an absorbing pigment around the rhabdom in bright light. This pigment absorbs light in eyes that have to function over a range of intensities. In dim light the pigment moves back, increasing the rhabdom's sensitivity and sometimes widening the ommatidium's field of view. In some insects adaptation to low light levels is achieved by the movement of the receptor toward the lens. Compound eyes that adapt to darkness in this way are known as mobile-cone (or acone) eyes;

they are found in hemipteran bugs, mosquitoes and some beetles.

Many nocturnal insects and some diurnal moths and beetles have superposition eyes with a quite different optical system, with the posterior nodal point at the center of curvature of the entire eye. The sensitivity of such eyes is increased by having the receptors close to the posterior nodal point. In still other insects the value of the eye parameter $D\Delta\phi$ at one position on the eye is quite different from the value at another position, suggesting that the eye is sensitive to a broad range of intensities. One can now see the value of knowing the eye parameter for any part of the compound eye before proceeding to study the eye in other ways.

For example, consider the eye of the housefly. When the eye parameter $D\Delta\phi$ measured from eye maps is compared with the ambient intensity of light at which the fly is usually active, one immediately sees what seems to be a discrepancy: the eye of the fly is apparently designed to operate at an ambient intensity some 10,000 times lower than that of full sunlight. The discrepancy is resolved when one remembers that flies not only prefer shady places but also use their eyes as they turn at high speed. High-speed maneuvers cause the environment to pass the eye at high angular

velocities, reducing the effective number of photons available to a photoreceptor. High-speed turns decrease the perceived intensity of the light by a factor of about 1,000. Such considerations have to do with why hover flies hover and perching dragonflies and the praying mantids remain motionless.

With the optics of the compound eye in mind one can turn to some maps of the eyes of insects prepared from measurements of the pseudopupil. Each circle on the eye maps has a diameter of $5\lambda/D$ radians, with the wavelength λ taken to be .5 micrometer (green light). Each circle represents the width of the blur circle of each fifth ommatidium. The size of the circles is thus the key to the local resolution of individual ommatidia: the smaller the circle, the better the resolution. The distance from the center of one circle to the center of the next is five times the interommatidial angle ($5\Delta\phi$). The proximity of the circles is a measure of the density with which the insect eye samples the visual world and so is a measure of the visual resolution in that region of the eye. The overlap of the circles shows the value of the eye parameter $D\Delta\phi$ at that place. For example, where the circles just touch, their diameter λ/D is equal to their separation $\Delta\phi$ and the eye parameter has a value of .5.

I have compiled maps of the eyes of representative types of insects and have found a number of general features.

First, there do not seem to be any insects whose eyes are designed primarily to operate near the diffraction limit. Earlier values suggesting that insect eyes are limited by diffraction are wrong. Even the eyes of the Australian sand wasp *Bembix,* which is active in the brilliant sunlight of the desert, have an eye parameter of .32 only in the center of the fovea. The eyes of mantids, which catch prey that are usually stationary in bright light, have an eye parameter that is surprisingly large, ranging between .5 and 2.

Second, most insects that fly in bright sunlight, such as bees, butterflies and dragonflies, have an eye parameter of about .5. This generalization should be applied with care, because a small change in the value of the eye parameter near that value implies a large difference in the optimum intensity at which the eye would function best.

Third, the eyes of carnivorous insects seem to have a larger eye parameter than the eyes of herbivorous insects in the same habitat, but the carnivorous insects also have foveas.

Fourth, it is common to find a smooth gradient in the value of the eye parameter horizontally across the eye of a single insect, from smaller values near the front of the eye to larger values around the side. Presumably the gradients in the eye parameter are related to the fact that when the insect is flying, objects at the side of the eye have a greater angular velocity and give rise to less modulation than objects in front of the eye. The gradients are best seen by following a horizontal row of facets in the eyes of locusts, hymenopterans and dragonflies, but they are also characteristic of mantids, ants and other insects that do not have horizontal rows of facets or rapid forward motion.

Fifth, along the equatorial region of the eye the pseudopupil is vertically elongated, because here the interommatidial angle between the facets in vertical rows is smaller than the interommatidial angle between the facets in horizontal ones. Although the apparent hexagonal pattern of the facets on the eye is little modified where the pseudopupil is

elongated, the optical axes of the facets are compressed in the vertical direction to form a diamond lattice, so that the eyes look out on the world from an array of oblique squares. As we have seen, such a square pattern enables the eye to sample the visual world more efficiently than a hexagonal pattern does. These considerations suggest the intriguing possibility that the eyes might use the vertical rows of ommatidia rather than the horizontal rows for tasks requiring high resolution.

Sixth, where there is much binocular overlap the eye is stretched over a wider total angle, and the eye parameter is then always larger than expected. This is the case in mantids and damselflies.

The eye maps also reveal much information about the foveas of insects.

First, a fovea is formed where rows of optical axes are gathered together, so that the density of ommatidia looking out is greater. A fovea is never formed by the interpolation of extra rows of ommatidia. The opposite is the case: in the foveal region rows of facets have to be left out to make room for the larger facets.

Second, the optical axes are gathered together by a warping of the rows of axes; the fact that the facets in a row are in a straight line does not necessarily indicate that their optical axes are lying in one plane.

Third, on the eye maps for some insect predators the circles of diameter λ/D overlap more in the fovea than they do in adjoining areas of the eye. This means that in the fovea the eye parame-

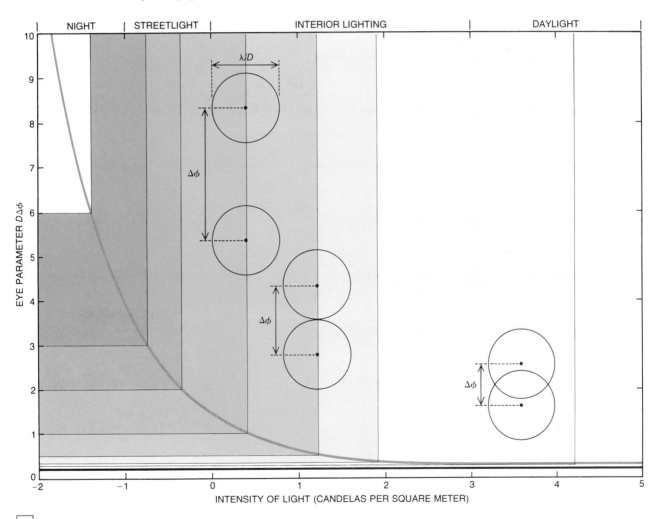

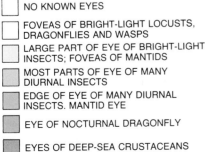

NO KNOWN EYES

FOVEAS OF BRIGHT-LIGHT LOCUSTS, DRAGONFLIES AND WASPS

LARGE PART OF EYE OF BRIGHT-LIGHT INSECTS; FOVEAS OF MANTIDS

MOST PARTS OF EYE OF MANY DIURNAL INSECTS

EDGE OF EYE OF MANY DIURNAL INSECTS. MANTID EYE

EYE OF NOCTURNAL DRAGONFLY

EYES OF DEEP-SEA CRUSTACEANS

EYE PARAMETER $D\Delta\phi$ (*curve in color*) **has a different optimum value for different levels of the ambient intensity of light. If the structure of the eyes of insects were determined only by the constraints of the diffraction of light, the eyes of all insects would have an eye parameter of approximately .25** (*horizontal line in black across the bottom*). **Circles of** λ/D **on the eye maps would then overlap halfway (not shown here). Instead only in the foveas of insects active in extremely bright sunlight does the eye parameter approach the diffraction limit** (*far right*). **Moreover, the eye of an insect frequently has different values of the eye parameter in different areas, apparently so that each area is most effective at the level of light intensity at which it is most used. A candela per square meter** (*horizontal axis*) **is a unit of luminous intensity.**

ter decreases, which in turn implies that in general the fovea is a region adapted for seeing in relatively bright light. In certain insects, however, such as the gomphid dragonfly *Austrogomphus,* the eye parameter remains constant across the fovea.

Fourth, the rows of facets are always more regular in the fovea than they are elsewhere on the eye, showing that regularity plays some important role in those regions of the eye where there is a need for the best possible seeing.

Fifth, although the facets in the fovea are usually larger than those elsewhere on the eye, that is not the case in the eyes of the locust *Locusta* and the mantid *Orthodera.* Both of those insects have a forward-looking fovea where the interommatidial angle is smaller but where the facets are the same size as those elsewhere on the eye. Such a fovea is perhaps a specialized area that enhances the visual acuity but has narrower and therefore less sensitive fields.

Sixth, in the sand wasp *Bembix,* which hovers to see in the extremely bright sunlight of the Australian desert, the eye parameter is as low as about .31 in the fovea, close to the diffraction limit. Many insects, however, have a remarkably large eye parameter even in the fovea. For example, the eye parameter reaches 1 in the fovea of the damselflies, which search for prey among reeds and under trees. Although in all cases the fovea is a region of higher visual resolution, it is clear that it can be a region of low sensitivity or can by having larger facets be designed to operate at the same intensity as the rest of the eye.

Although it must be true that the visual habits of insects are written on their eyeballs, it is difficult to read the signs correctly because we know so little about how the eyes are used. Presumably eyes that look sideways, such as those of some birds or of the rabbit, are early-warning devices. A clue is provided by locusts and flies, which are very sensitive to movement at the side of the head and are relatively insensitive to movement at the front. The large lateral fovea that looks directly sideways in many large dragonflies is puzzling; possibly it helps the animal to hover over water. The interommatidial angles between the facets of that fovea are less than .5 degree, the smallest I have found in any insect.

Insects that hunt visually would presumably need a forward-looking fovea. There is still some doubt, however, about whether most insect foveas, like those of vertebrates, work better in brighter light. If they do, then dragonflies, hunting wasps and mantids may suffer a decrease in visual acuity at dusk, much as human beings do.

The eyes of mantids are puzzling in many ways. In most mantids the fovea is quite obvious. Yet in 1971 J. C. Barros-Pita and H. Maldonado in Venezuela showed that the area immediately surrounding the fovea as it is defined here (not the center of the fovea) is the area that is essential in enabling the insect to see well enough to catch prey. Moreover, out of a large selection of mantids for which I have made eye maps none had circles of λ/D that overlapped outside the fovea region. Even more remarkable, the eyes of the largest mantids, which have facets as much as 50 micrometers across at the center of the fovea, have an eye parameter elsewhere greater than 2; thus the center-to-center separation of the circles on the eye maps is more than twice their diameter of λ/D. The only available explanation is that the mantid eye has 45 degrees of binocular overlap on each eye, so that the

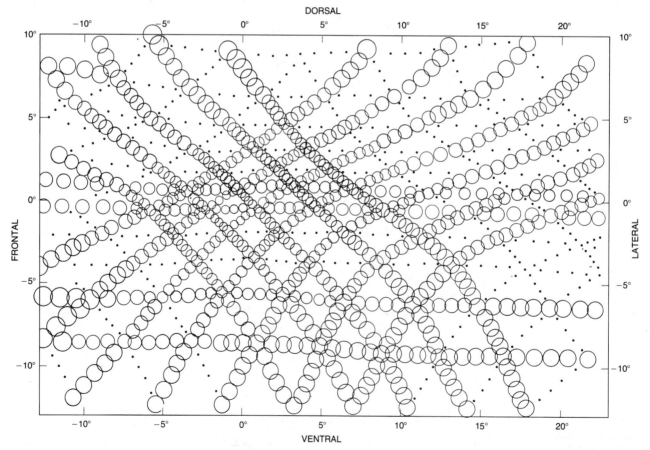

EYE MAP OF SAND WASP *Bembix palmata* reveals that the optical axes of the insect's ommatidia (*dots and centers of circles*) do not follow the same hexagonal pattern that its eye facets do. Along the horizontal axis of the map they are in a pattern of oblique squares that become more oblique toward the equator of the eye. The circles have a diameter of λ/D. The large overlap between them indicates that the eye parameter is about .3. *Bembix* is one of the few insects for which the eye parameter (and then only the parameter in the fovea near 0 degrees, 0 degrees in angle coordinates) very nearly approaches the diffraction limit. *Bembix* is active in the brilliant sunlight of the Australian desert, so that photon noise is low with respect to intensity of the light and the diffraction limit can be approached.

eyes are stretched over an abnormally wide visual world.

At first the fact that dragonflies have foveas that look obliquely forward and upward is also puzzling. It may be relevant, however, that a helicopter flying at full speed tilts forward so that the lift of its rotating blades is also the forward thrust. Dragonflies have some resemblance to helicopters, and it is possible that their upward-looking foveas are actually looking straight at the prey they are pursuing in the air. Moreover, an upward-looking fovea is exactly what an insect needs in order to anticipate the position of a falling object or to approach prey from below. In addition the top of the dragonfly eye is predominantly sensitive to short wavelengths of light, which suggests that the eye perceives the highest contrast and has the best resolution when it is looking at objects against the blue of the sky.

The theoretical relation between the value of the eye parameter and the effective intensity of light at which each part of the compound eye must function serves to bring together a vast amount of data. The theory is underlain by three basic assumptions: first, that the compound eye is an array of receptors that processes information simultaneously through parallel channels; second, that the facets and rhabdoms of the eye must be large enough to catch a sufficient number of photons to perceive the modulation above the noise, and third, that a striped pattern resolved by any single receptor can also be seen as a pattern by the eye as a whole.

From a survey of studies of insect vision one might raise the objection that there is little evidence the last assumption is true, or that a fine pattern is in fact reconstructed by any compound eye. Such evidence does, however, exist. First, numerous tests with bees that have been trained to respond to patterns show that two aspects of the pattern are important to a bee: the amount of flicker the pattern creates as it sweeps across the compound eyes and the angles and colors of the pattern's contrasting edges. Patterns that look very different to the human eye are readily confused by the trained bee if the patterns cause similar amounts of flicker. Second, for an insect to perceive the speed and direction of a pattern moving across its eye the most important aspect of the signal is not the pattern itself but the sequential appearance of the signal at successive visual axes across the eye.

It is difficult to devise an experiment that will conclusively test whether or not an insect reconstitutes a pattern in its brain and thus perceives it as an actual pattern. It is easy to demonstrate, however, that an insect can respond to a very small movement of a large object and that it will respond particularly well to a small movement of a small object. In

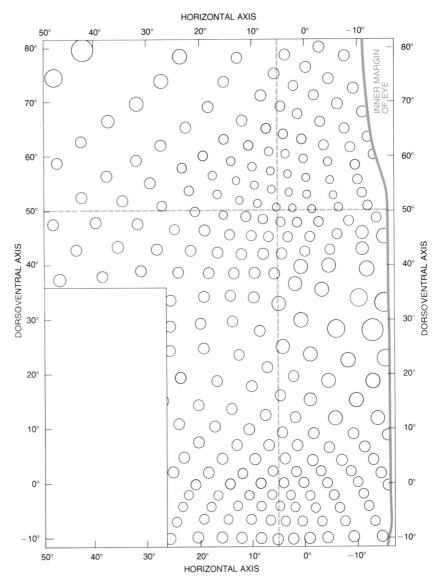

EYE MAP OF NOCTURNAL DRAGONFLY *Zyxomma* shows the optical axis of every fifth ommatidium. *Zyxomma*, an insect of Southeast Asia, comes out to feed only at twilight. The map shows the extreme separation of the circles (of diameters $5\lambda/D$ radians), the shallow fovea of the insect's eye looking obliquely forward and upward near 0 degrees, 50 degrees on the axes, and crowding of axes along horizontal zero axis (*bottom of map*). Broken lines show lines along which there are no errors due to mapping of curved surface of insect eye on a flat sheet.

many small insects, which do not have room in their head for large eyes, the interommatidial angle can be as large as 10 degrees, yet a number of careful studies have shown that those insects can respond to detail subtending an angle as small as a tenth of the interommatidial angle. Part of the secret possibly lies in the fact that some insects may make use of eye tremor to scan the visual world and sequentially build up a more detailed picture of it as a pattern in time instead of in space. That would go against the assumption that sampling must be simultaneous.

To some extent the objections that can be raised against the assumptions underlying the optical theory I have discussed here cancel one another. For example, seeing motion requires that the insect be sensitive to the exact timing of small modulations at each visual axis over a region of the eye. Seeing the direction of a contrasting edge requires that the insect be sensitive to the exact phase of the sinusoidal (striped) components of the pattern. Seeing the relative movement of a small dark object in an unpredictable direction against a complex dappled background that is also moving, as a flying insect hunting for prey surely does, requires all the information the eye can get. I suspect that as we examine the visual behavior of insects more closely we shall find that there is a premium on gathering all possible information. The form of the most advanced compound eyes suggests that they are designed to collect the maximum amount of information they possibly can in a continuing battle against photon noise.

II

PATHWAYS TO THE MIND'S EYE

II PATHWAYS TO THE MIND'S EYE

INTRODUCTION

Before anything resembling perception can occur, the visual system must extract from its input the location and orientation of edges. It has to measure velocities, identify colors, and so on. A combination of anatomical, physiological, and psychophysical data shows us that this "feature extraction" is done by specialized mechanisms, or "channels," one "set" of channels for each feature. A set of channels to identify the precise orientation of a contour, for example, might include a channel for horizontal contours, one for contours tilted 30 degrees from the vertical, and so on.

The physiological and anatomical work that won Hubel and Wiesel the Nobel prize in 1981 is a good starting point for an understanding of these mechanisms. These two scientists and others have examined the responses of single cells in the visual pathways of cats and monkeys. In the retina, cells respond to spots of light or dark. The same is true at the first stop along the visual pathway in the brain, the lateral geniculate nucleus of the thalamus. However, at the next major stop, the primary visual cortex, cells are optimally stimulated by the orientation of an object and by motion in specific directions.

The visual cortex is a very orderly structure. Cells in one region of cortex respond to light from one region of visual space. In a neighboring region of cortex, cells respond to stimuli in a neighboring region of space. Within a region (or "hypercolumn") there is further differentiation. For example, if we move vertically down into the cortex, all of the cells will be most strongly activated by lines of the same (or similar) orientation. As we move to one side, this preferred orientation will change systematically. The whole range of possible orientations will be represented within one hypercolumn.

Of course, most of the methods used in studies with animals cannot be applied to human subjects. We must use "psychophysical" methods to study feature extraction in humans. By presenting subjects with stimuli and measuring their responses, we can make "inferences" about the processes going on inside their inaccessible brains.

The phenomenon of negative aftereffects, as discussed by Favreau, is a good example of a powerful psychophysical tool. Brain cells, like muscle cells, become fatigued with use. Suppose you stare at a red light. The cells that are most activated by red will become fatigued and will respond less briskly. If you were to look at a white light after staring at the red one, the white light would appear blue-green. White light normally activates all of the color-sensitive cells, but when fatigued, the red-sensitive cells are inactive compared to the cells that respond best to blue and green. Similar effects occur in the perception of motion, size, orientation, and so forth.

There is a good correspondence between the stimuli that can produce aftereffects and the basic features that are extracted by the visual cortex.

While it makes sense to regard many aftereffects as by-products of fatigue of the feature-extracting mechanisms, there is a complication—some aftereffects last for a very long time. Favreau discusses the McCollough effect, which can last for months, far longer than any plausible fatigue. The long-lasting effects change the way we see such things as "white," "stationary," or "vertical." Consider the example of "stationary." The eye is always moving. Even when one tries to hold a fixed gaze, there is a tremor. What then is stationary? There are no external stimuli that form stationary images on the retina. The visual system must "learn" the definition of stationary (and of white, vertical, and so on). Long-term aftereffects may be a result of that learning process.

In the Sekuler and Levinson article, the phenomenon of aftereffects and other psychophysical methods are used to explore the processing of motion information. In addition to describing the extraction of one visual feature, this article demonstrates that our ability to see a complex stimulus can be understood in terms of our ability to see its simpler components. The authors' example is a "counterphased" grating, a flickering pattern that is treated by the visual system as the sum of two sets of moving bars.

In the final article in this section, I use another variation on the aftereffect method to uncover some of the details of binocular visual processing; in this case, a binocular process that is active only if the left and right eye are stimulated at the same time by the same thing. The remainder of my article deals with visual pathways that do not lead to the "mind's eye." They are involved in such activities as controlling eye movement or focussing the eyes. For example, your ability to focus is controlled by processes that are entirely color-blind. Although you can read about the experiments that prove this, you can never directly experience this color blindness nor, for that matter, can you directly experience the automatic extraction of features such as size or color, even though it occurs in the main visual pathway.

To summarize this section, the path from the eye to the mind's eye involves the extraction of a limited number of basic features (motion, orientation, color, etc.) from visual input. Because we cannot consciously examine the function of our own feature extractors, we must study them with psychophysical methods. Finally, it is important to remember that we have several parallel visual pathways, and that what we see is just one of the results of visual processing.

4

Brain Mechanisms of Vision

by David H. Hubel and Torsten N. Wiesel
September 1979

A functional architecture that may underlie processing of sensory information in the cortex is revealed by studies of the activity and the organization in space of neurons in the primary visual cortex

Viewed as a kind of invention by evolution, the cerebral cortex must be one of the great success stories in the history of living things. In vertebrates lower than mammals the cerebral cortex is minuscule, if it can be said to exist at all. Suddenly impressive in the lowest mammals, it begins to dominate the brain in carnivores, and it increases explosively in primates; in man it almost completely envelops the rest of the brain, tending to obscure the other parts. The degree to which an animal depends on an organ is an index of the organ's importance that is even more convincing than size, and dependence on the cortex has increased rapidly as mammals have evolved. A mouse without a cortex appears fairly normal, at least to casual inspection; a man without a cortex is almost a vegetable, speechless, sightless, senseless.

Understanding of this large and indispensable organ is still woefully deficient. This is partly because it is very complex, not only structurally but also in its functions, and partly because neurobiologists' intuitions about the functions have so often been wrong. The outlook is changing, however, as techniques improve and as investigators learn how to deal with the huge numbers of intricately connected neurons that are the basic elements of the cortex, with the impulses they carry and with the synapses that connect them. In this article we hope to sketch the present state of knowledge of one subdivision of the cortex: the primary visual cortex (also known as the striate cortex or area 17), the most elementary of the cortical regions concerned with vision. That will necessarily lead us into the related subject of visual perception, since the workings of an organ cannot easily be separated from its biological purpose.

The cerebral cortex, a highly folded plate of neural tissue about two millimeters thick, is an outermost crust wrapped over the top of, and to some extent tucked under, the cerebral hemispheres. In man its total area, if it were spread out, would be about 1.5 square feet. (In a 1963 article in *Scientific American* one of us gave the area as 20 square feet and was quickly corrected by a neuroanatomist friend in Toronto, who said he thought it was 1.5 square feet—"at least that is what Canadians have.") The folding is presumably mainly the result of such an unlikely structure's having to be packed into a box the size of the skull.

A casual glance at cortical tissue under a microscope shows vast numbers of neurons: about 10^5 (100,000) for each square millimeter of surface, suggesting that the cortex as a whole has some 10^{10} (10 billion) neurons. The cell bodies are arranged in half a dozen layers that are alternately cell-sparse and cell-rich. In contrast to these marked changes in cell density in successive layers at different depths in the cortex there is marked uniformity from place to place in the plane of any given layer and in any direction within that plane. The cortex is morphologically rather uniform in two of its dimensions.

One of the first great insights about cortical organization came late in the 19th century, when it was gradually realized that this rather uniform plate of tissue is subdivided into a number of different regions that have very different functions. The evidence came from clinical, physiological and anatomical sources. It was noted that a brain injury, depending on its location, could cause paralysis or blindness or numbness or speech loss; the blindness could be total or limited to half or less of the visual world, and the numbness could involve one limb or a few fingers. The consistency of the relation between a given defect and the location of the lesion gradually led to a charting of the most obvious of these specialized regions, the visual, auditory, somatic sensory (body sensation), speech and motor regions.

In many cases a close look with a microscope at cortex stained for cell bodies showed that in spite of the relative uniformity there were structural variations, particularly in the layering pattern, that correlated well with the clinically defined subdivisions. Additional confirmation came from observations of the location (at the surface of the brain) of the electrical brain waves produced when an animal was stimulated by touching the body, sounding clicks or tones in the ear or flashing light in the eye. Similarly, motor areas could be mapped by stimulating the cortex electrically and noting what part of the animal's body moved.

This systematic mapping of the cortex soon led to a fundamental realization: most of the sensory and motor areas contained systematic two-dimensional maps of the world they represented. Destroying a particular small region of cortex could lead to paralysis of one arm; a similar lesion in another small region led to numbness of one hand or of the upper lip, or blindness in one small part of the visual world; if electrodes were placed on an animal's cortex, touching one limb produced a correspondingly localized series of electric potentials. Clearly the body was systematically mapped onto the somatic sensory and motor areas; the visual world was mapped onto the primary visual cortex, an area on the occipital lobe that in man and in the macaque monkey (the animal in which our investigations have mainly been conducted) covers about 15 square centimeters.

In the primary visual cortex the map is uncomplicated by breaks and discontinuities except for the remarkable split of the visual world down the exact middle, with the left half projected to the right cerebral cortex and the right half projected to the left cortex. The map of the body is more complicated and is still perhaps not completely understood. It is nonetheless systematic, and it is similarly crossed, with the right side of the body projecting to the left hemisphere and the left side projecting to the right hemisphere. (It is worth remarking that no one has the remotest idea why there should be this amazing tendency for nervous-system pathways to cross.)

An important feature of cortical maps is their distortion. The scale of the maps varies as it does in a Mercator projection, the rule for the cortex being that

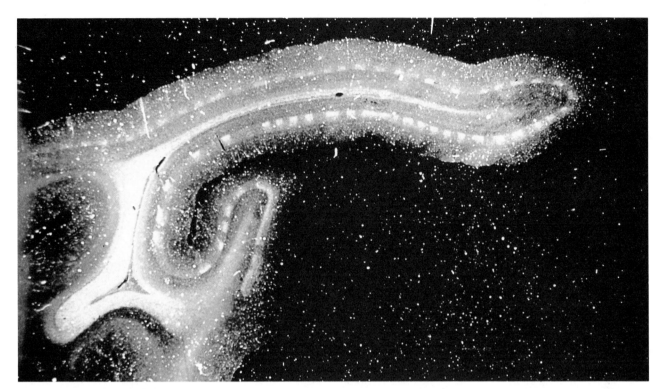

OCULAR-DOMINANCE COLUMNS, one of the two major systems that characterize the functional architecture of the primary visual cortex, are revealed as periodic bright patches in this dark-field autoradiograph of a section of macaque monkey cortex. The columns (actually curving slabs of cortex, seen here in cross section in a brain slice cut perpendicularly to the surface) are regions in which all neurons respond more actively to the right eye than to the left one; dark regions separating the bright patches are columns of left-eye prefer-ence. The autoradiograph was made by injecting a radioactively labeled amino acid into the right eye of an anesthetized animal. The amino acid was taken up by cell bodies in the retina and transport-ed via the lateral geniculate nucleus, a way station in the brain, to cells in the cortex. A brain slice was coated with a photographic emul-sion, which was exposed for several months and then developed. Ex-posed silver grains overlying the regions of radioactivity form the light-scattering patches that represent ocular-dominance columns.

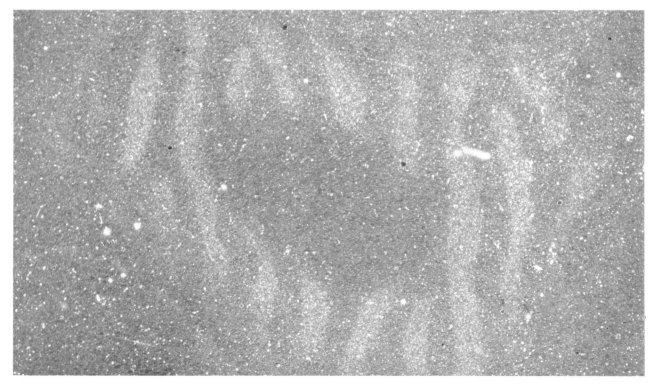

DOMINANCE PATTERN is seen face on in an axonal-transport autoradiograph of a brain section parallel, rather than perpendicu-lar, to the surface of the primary visual cortex. As can be seen in the autoradiograph at the top of the page, the label is brightest in one layer of the folded cortex, layer IV. This is the level at which the ax-ons bringing visual information to the cortex terminate and where the label therefore accumulates. This section was cut in a plane tan-gential to the dome-shaped surface of the cortex and just below lay-er IV, which therefore appears as a ring of roughly parallel bright bands. These are the radioactively labeled ocular-dominance regions, which are now seen from above instead of edge on. The actual width of the ocular-dominance regions is typically about .4 millimeter.

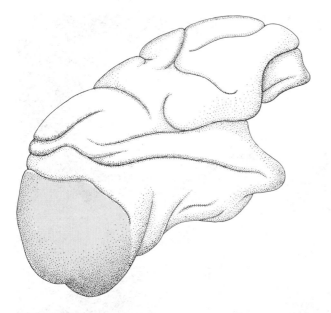

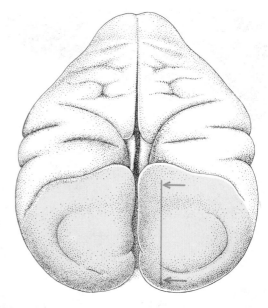

PRIMARY VISUAL CORTEX, also known as the striate cortex or area 17, is a region of the cerebral cortex: a layered plate of neurons that envelops the primate brain. In the macaque brain, seen here from the side (*left*) and from above and behind (*right*), the primary visual cortex (*colored areas*) occupies most of the exposed surface of **the two occipital lobes. It also curves around the medial surface between the two cerebral hemispheres. It continues in a complex fold underneath the convex outer surface, as is shown in a parasagittal section (*see top illustration on opposite page*) that was cut along the colored line and is viewed in the direction indicated by the arrows.**

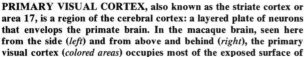

the regions of highest discrimination or delicacy of function occupy relatively more cortical area. For the body surface, a millimeter of surface on the fingers, the lips or the tongue projects to more cortex than a millimeter of trunk, buttocks or back; in vision the central part of the retina has a representation some 35 times more detailed than the far peripheral part.

Important as the advances in mapping cortical projections were, they tended for some time to divert thought from the real problem of just how the brain analyzes information. It was as though the representation could be an end in itself instead of serving a more subtle purpose—as though what the cortex did was to cater to some little green man who sat inside the head and surveyed images playing across the cortex. In the course of this article we shall show that, for vision at least, the world is represented in a far more distorted way; any little green man trying to glean information from the cortical projection would be puzzled indeed.

The first major insight into cortical organization was nonetheless the recognition of this subdivision into areas having widely different functions, with a tendency to ordered mapping. Just how many such areas there are has been a subject of wide speculation. Anatomists' estimates have on the whole been rather high—up to several hundred areas, depending on the individual worker's sensitivity to fine differences in microscopic patterns and sometimes also on his ability to fool himself. Physiologists began with lower estimates, but lately, with more powerful mapping methods, they

have been revising their estimates upward. The important basic notion is that information on any given modality such as sight or sound is transmitted first to a primary cortical area and from there, either directly or via the thalamus, to successions of higher areas. A modern guess as to the number of cortical areas might be between 50 and 100.

The second major insight into cortical organization came from the work of the anatomist Santiago Ramón y Cajal and his pupil Rafael Lorente de Nó. This was the realization that the operations the cortex performs on the information it receives are local. What that means can best be understood by considering the wiring diagram that emerged from the Golgi method used by Cajal and Lorente de Nó. In essence the wiring is simple. Sets of fibers bring information to the cortex; by the time several synapses have been traversed the influence of the input has spread vertically to all cell layers; finally several other sets of fibers carry modified messages out of the area. The detailed connections between inputs and outputs differ from one area to the next, but within a given area they seem to be rather stereotyped. What is common to all regions is the local nature of the wiring. The information carried into the cortex by a single fiber can in principle make itself felt through the entire thickness in about three or four synapses, whereas the lateral spread, produced by branching trees of axons and dendrites, is limited for all practical purposes to a few millimeters, a small proportion of the vast extent of the cortex.

The implications of this are far-reaching. Whatever any given region of the cortex does, it does locally. At stages where there is any kind of detailed, systematic topographical mapping the analysis must be piecemeal. For example, in the somatic sensory cortex the messages concerning one finger can be combined and compared with an input from elsewhere on that same finger or with input from a neighboring finger, but they can hardly be combined with the influence from the trunk or from a foot. The same applies to the visual world. Given the detailed order of the input to the primary visual cortex, there is no likelihood that the region will do anything to correlate information coming in from both far above and far below the horizon, or from both the left and the right part of the visual scene. It follows that this cannot by any stretch of the imagination be the place where actual perception is enshrined. Whatever these cortical areas are doing, it must be some kind of local analysis of the sensory world. One can only assume that as the information on vision or touch or sound is relayed from one cortical area to the next the map becomes progressively more blurred and the information carried more abstract.

Even though the Golgi-method studies of the early 1900's made it clear that the cortex must perform local analyses, it was half a century before physiologists had the least inkling of just what the analysis was in any area of the cortex. The first understanding came in the primary visual area, which is now the best-understood of any cortical region and is still the only one where the analysis and consequent transformations of information are known in any detail. After describing the main transformations that take place in the primary visual cortex we shall go on to show how increasing understanding of these cortical functions has revealed an entire world of architectural order that is otherwise inaccessible to observation.

We can best begin by tracing the visual path in a primate from the retina to the cortex. The output from each eye is conveyed to the brain by about a million nerve fibers bundled together in the optic nerve. These fibers are the axons of the ganglion cells of the retina. The messages from the light-sensitive elements, the rods and cones, have already traversed from two to four synapses and have involved four other types of retinal cells before they arrive at the ganglion cells, and a certain amount of sophisticated analysis of the information has already taken place.

A large fraction of the optic-nerve fibers pass uninterrupted to two nests of cells deep in the brain called the lateral geniculate nuclei, where they make synapses. The lateral geniculate cells in turn send their axons directly to the primary visual cortex. From there, after several synapses, the messages are sent to a number of further destinations: neighboring cortical areas and also several targets deep in the brain. One contingent even projects back to the lateral geniculate bodies; the function of this feedback path is not known. The main point for the moment is that the primary visual cortex is in no sense the end of the visual path. It is just one stage, probably an early one in terms of the degree of abstraction of the information it handles.

As a result of the partial crossing of the optic nerves in the optic chiasm, the geniculate and the cortex on the left side are connected to the two left half retinas and are therefore concerned with the right half of the visual scene, and the converse is the case for the right geniculate and the right cortex. Each geniculate and each cortex receives input from both eyes, and each is concerned with the opposite half of the visual world.

To examine the workings of this visual pathway our strategy since the late 1950's has been (in principle) simple. Beginning, say, with the fibers of the optic nerve, we record with microelectrodes from a single nerve fiber and try to find out how we can most effectively influence the firing by stimulating the retina with light. For this one can use patterns of light of every conceivable size, shape and color, bright on a dark background or the reverse, and stationary or moving. It may take a long time, but sooner or later we satisfy ourselves that we have found the best stimulus for the cell being tested, in this case a ganglion cell of the retina. (Sometimes we are

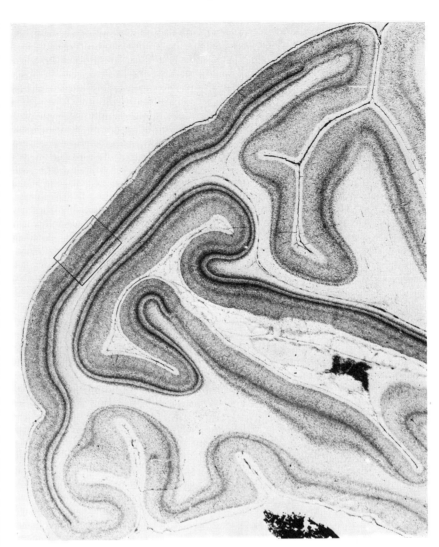

SECTION OF VISUAL CORTEX along the colored line in the illustration on the opposite page was stained by the Nissl method, which makes cell bodies but not fibers visible. The visual cortex is seen to be a continuous layered sheet of neurons about two millimeters thick. The black rectangle outlines a section like the one that is further enlarged in the illustration below.

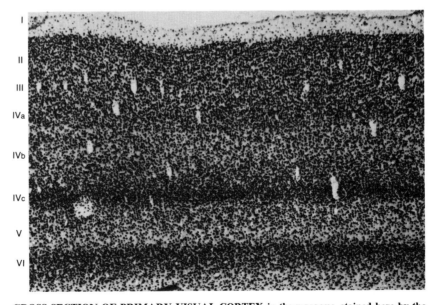

CROSS SECTION OF PRIMARY VISUAL CORTEX in the macaque, stained here by the Nissl method and enlarged about 35 diameters, shows the layered structure and gives the conventional designations of the six layers (*left*). The white gaps are sectioned blood vessels.

wrong!) We note the results and then go on to another fiber. After studying a few hundred cells we may find that new types become rare. Satisfied that we know roughly how the neurons at this stage work, we proceed to the next stage (in this case the geniculate) and repeat the process. Comparison of the two sets of results can tell us something about what the geniculate does. We then go on to the next stage, the primary cortex, and repeat the procedure.

Working in this way, one finds that both a retinal ganglion cell and a geniculate cell respond best to a roughly circular spot of light of a particular size in a particular part of the visual field. The size is critical because each cell's receptive field (the patch of retinal receptor cells supplying the cell) is divided, with an excitatory center and an inhibitory surround (an "on center" cell) or exactly the reverse configuration (an "off center" cell). This is the center-surround configuration first described by Stephen W. Kuffler at the Johns Hopkins University School of Medicine in 1953. A spot exactly filling the center of an on-center cell is therefore a more effective stimulus than a larger spot that invades the inhibitory area, or than diffuse light. A line stimulus (a bar of light) is effective if it covers a large part of the center region and only a small part of the surround. Because these cells have circular symmetry they respond well to such a line stimulus whatever its orientation. To sum up, the retinal ganglion cells and the cells of the lateral geniculate—the cells supplying the input to the visual cortex—are cells with concentric, center-surround receptive fields. They are primarily concerned not with assessing levels of illumination but rather with making a comparison between the light level in one small area of the visual scene and the average illumination of the immediate surround.

The first of the two major transformations accomplished by the visual cortex is the rearrangement of incoming information so that most of its cells respond not to spots of light but to specifically oriented line segments. There is a wide variety of cell types in the cortex, some simpler and some more complex in their response properties, and one soon gains an impression of a kind of hierarchy, with simpler cells feeding more complex ones. In the monkey there is first of all a large group of cells that behave (as far as is known) just like geniculate cells: they have circularly symmetrical fields. These cells are all in the lower part of one layer, called layer IV, which is precisely the layer that receives the lion's share of the geniculate input. It makes sense that these least sophisticated cortical cells should be the ones most immediately connected to the input.

Cells outside layer IV all respond best to specifically oriented line segments. A typical cell responds only when light falls in a particular part of the visual world, but illuminating that area diffusely has little effect or none, and small spots of light are not much better. The best response is obtained when a line that has just the right tilt is flashed in the region or, in some cells, is swept across the region. The most effective orientation varies from cell to cell and is usually defined sharply enough so that a change of 10 or 20 degrees clockwise or counterclockwise reduces the response markedly or abolishes it. (It is hard to convey the precision of this discrimination. If 10 to 20 degrees sounds like a wide range, one should remember that the angle between 12 o'clock and one o'clock is 30 degrees.) A line at 90 degrees to the best orientation almost never evokes any response.

Depending on the particular cell, the stimulus may be a bright line on a dark background or the reverse, or it may be a boundary between light and dark regions. If it is a line, the thickness is likely to be important; increasing it beyond some optimal width reduces the response, just as increasing the diameter of a spot does in the case of ganglion and geniculate cells. Indeed, for a particular part of the visual field the geniculate receptive-field centers and the optimal cortical line widths are comparable.

Neurons with orientation specificity vary in their complexity. The simplest, which we call "simple" cells, behave as though they received their input directly from several cells with center-surround, circularly symmetrical fields—the type of cells found in layer IV. The response properties of these simple cells, which respond to an optimally oriented line in a narrowly defined location, can most easily be accounted for by requiring that the centers of the incoming center-surround fields all be excitatory or all be inhibitory, and that they lie along a straight line. At present we have no direct evidence for this scheme, but it is attractive because of its simplicity and because certain kinds of indirect evidence support it. According to the work of Jennifer S. Lund of the University of Washington School of Medicine, who in the past few years has done more than anyone else to advance the Golgi-stain anatomy of this cortical area, the cells in layer IV project to the layers just above, which is roughly where the simple cells are found.

The second major group of orientation-specific neurons are the far more numerous "complex" cells. They come in a number of subcategories, but their main feature is that they are less particular about the exact position of a line.

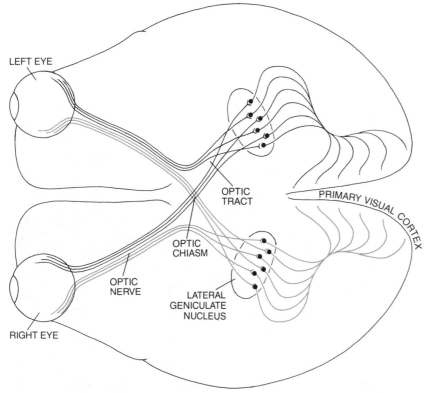

LEFT EYE

OPTIC TRACT

PRIMARY VISUAL CORTEX

OPTIC CHIASM

OPTIC NERVE

LATERAL GENICULATE NUCLEUS

RIGHT EYE

VISUAL PATHWAY is traced schematically in the human brain, seen here from below. The output from the retina is conveyed, by ganglion-cell axons bundled in the optic nerves, to the lateral geniculate nuclei; about half of the axons cross over to the opposite side of the brain, so that a representation of each half of the visual scene is projected on the geniculate of the opposite hemisphere. Neurons in the geniculates send their axons to the primary visual cortex.

RIGHT EYE

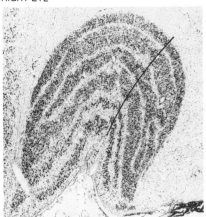

LEFT EYE

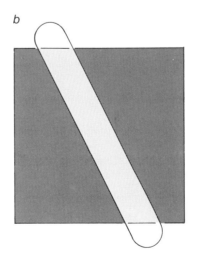

RIGHT EYE

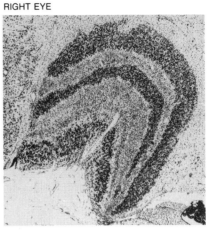

LATERAL GENICULATE NUCLEUS of a normal monkey (*left*) is a layered structure in which cells in layers 1, 4 and 6 (numbered from bottom to top) receive their input from the eye on the opposite side and those in layers 2, 3 and 5 receive information from the eye on the same side. The maps are in register, so that the neurons along any radius (*black line*) receive signals from the same part of the visual scene. The layered nature of the input is demonstrated in the two geniculates of an animal that had vision in the left eye only (*two micrographs at right*): in each geniculate cells in the three layers with input from right eye have atrophied. Geniculates are enlarged 10 diameters.

Complex cells behave as though they received their input from a number of simple cells, all with the same receptive-field orientation but differing slightly in the exact location of their fields. This scheme readily explains the strong steady firing evoked in a complex cell as a line is kept in the optimal orientation and is swept across the receptive field. With the line optimally oriented many cells prefer one direction of movement to the opposite direction. Several possible circuits have been proposed to explain this behavior, but the exact mechanism is still not known.

Although there is no direct evidence that orientation-sensitive cells have anything to do with visual perception, it is certainly tempting to think they represent some early stage in the brain's analysis of visual forms. It is worth asking which cells at this early stage would be expected to be turned on by some very simple visual form, say a dark blob on a light background. Any cell whose receptive field is entirely inside or outside the boundaries of such an image will be completely unaffected by the figure's presence because cortical cells effectively ignore diffuse changes in the illumination of their entire receptive fields.

The only cells to be affected will be those whose field is cut by the borders. For the circularly symmetrical cells the ones most strongly influenced will be those whose center is grazed by a boundary (because for them the excitatory and inhibitory subdivisions are most unequally illuminated). For the orientation-specific cells the only ones to be activated will be those whose optimal orientation happens to coincide with the prevailing direction of the border. And among these the simple cells will be much more exacting than the complex ones, responding optimally only when the border falls along a line separating an excitatory and an inhibitory region. It is important to realize that this part of the cortex is operating only locally, on bits of the form; how the entire form is analyzed or handled by the brain—how this information is worked on and synthesized at later stages, if indeed it is—is still not known.

The second major function of the monkey visual cortex is to combine the inputs from the two eyes. In the lateral geniculate nuclei a neuron may re-

a

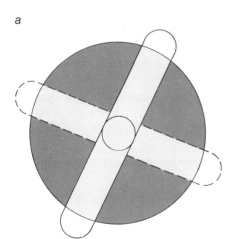

b

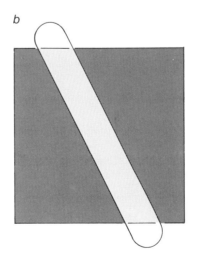

c

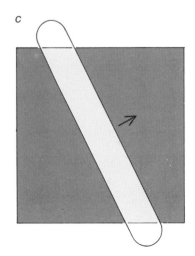

RECEPTIVE FIELDS of various cells in the visual pathway are compared. Retinal ganglion cells and neurons in the lateral geniculate nucleus have circular fields with either an excitatory center and an inhibitory surround (*a*) or the opposite arrangement. A spot of light falling on the center stimulates a response from such a cell; so does a bar of light falling on the field in any orientation, provided it falls on the center. In the visual cortex there is a hierarchy of neurons with increasingly complex response properties. The cortical cells that receive signals directly from the geniculate have circularly symmetrical fields. Cortical cells farther along the pathway, however, respond only to a line stimulus in a particular orientation. A "simple" cell (*b*) responds to such a line stimulus only in a particular part of its field. A "complex" cell (*c*) responds to a precisely oriented line regardless of where it is in its field and also to one moving in a particular direction (*arrow*).

spond to stimulation of the left eye or of the right one, but no cell responds to stimulation of both eyes. This may seem surprising, since each geniculate receives inputs from both eyes, but the fact is that the geniculates are constructed in a way that keeps inputs from the two eyes segregated. Each geniculate body is divided into six layers, three left-eye layers interdigitated with three right-eye ones. The opposite-side half of the visual world is mapped onto each layer (with the six maps in precise register, so that in a radial pathway traversing the six layers the receptive fields of all the cells encountered have virtually identical positions in the visual field). Since any one layer has input from only one eye, the individual cells of that layer must be monocular.

Even in the visual cortex the neurons to which the geniculate cells project directly, the circularly symmetrical cells in layer IV, are all (as far as we can tell) strictly monocular; so are all the simple cells. Only at the level of the complex cells do the paths from the two eyes converge, and even there the blending of information is incomplete and takes a special form. About half of the complex cells are monocular, in the sense that any one cell can be activated only by stimulating one eye. The rest of the cells can be influenced independently by both eyes.

If one maps the right-eye and left-eye receptive fields of a binocular cell (by stimulating first through one eye and then through the other) and compares the two fields, the fields turn out to have identical positions, levels of complexity, orientation and directional preference; everything one learns about the cell by stimulating one eye is confirmed through the other eye. There is only one exception: if first one eye and then the other are tested with identical stimuli, the two responses are usually not quantitatively identical; in many cases one eye is dominant, consistently producing a higher frequency of firing than the other eye.

From cell to cell all degrees of ocular dominance can be found, from complete monopoly by one eye through equality to exclusive control by the other eye. In the monkey the cells with a marked eye preference are somewhat commoner than the cells in which the two eyes make about equal contributions. Apparently a binocular cell in the primary visual cortex has connections to the two eyes that are qualitatively virtually identical, but the density of the two sets of connections is not necessarily the same.

It is remarkable enough that the elaborate sets of wiring that produce specificity of orientation and of direction of movement and other special properties

should be present in two duplicate copies. It is perhaps even more surprising that all of this can be observed in a newborn animal. The wiring is mostly innate, and it presumably is genetically determined. (In one particular respect, however, some maturation of binocular wiring does take place mostly after birth.)

We now turn to a consideration of the way these cells are grouped in the cortex. Are cells with similar characteristics—complexity, receptive-field position, orientation and ocular dominance—grouped together or scattered at random? From the description so far it will be obvious that cells of like complexity tend to be grouped in layers, with the circularly symmetrical cells low in layer IV, the simple cells just above them and the complex cells in layers II, III, V and VI. Complex cells can be further subcategorized, and the ones found in each layer are in a number of ways very different.

These differences from layer to layer take on added interest in view of the important discovery, confirmed by several physiologists and anatomists during the past few decades, that fibers projecting from particular layers of the cortex have particular destinations. For example, in the visual cortex the deepest layer, layer VI, projects mainly (perhaps only) back to the lateral geniculate body; layer V projects to the superior colliculus, a visual station in the midbrain; layers II and III send their projections to other parts of the cortex. This relation between layer and projection site probably deserves to be ranked as a third major insight into cortical organization.

The next stimulus variable to be considered is the position of the receptive field in the visual field. In describing the lateral geniculate nucleus we pointed out that in each layer the opposite-half visual field forms an ordered topographical map. In the projection from lateral geniculate to primary visual cortex this order is preserved, producing a cortical map of the visual field. Given this ordered map it is no surprise that neighboring cells in this part of the cortex always have receptive fields that are close together; usually, in fact, they overlap. If one plunges a microelectrode into the cortex at a right angle to the surface and records from cell after cell (as many as 100 or 200 of them) in successively deeper layers, again the receptive fields mostly overlap, with each new field heaped on all the others. The extent of the entire pile of fields is usually several times the size of any one typical field.

There is some variation in the size of these receptive fields. Some of the variation is tied to the layering: the largest fields in any penetration tend to be in

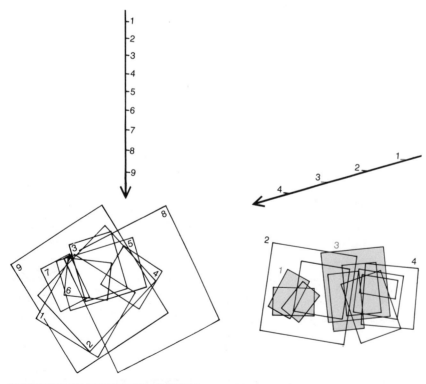

POSITIONS OF RECEPTIVE FIELDS (*numbered from 1 to 9*) of cortical neurons mapped by an electrode penetrating at roughly a right angle to the surface are essentially the same (*left*), although the fields are different sizes and there is some scatter. In an oblique penetration (*right*) from two to four cells were recorded, at .1-millimeter intervals, at each of four sites (*numbered from 1 to 4*) one millimeter apart. Each group includes various sizes and some scatter, but now there is also a systematic drift: fields of each successive group of cells are somewhat displaced.

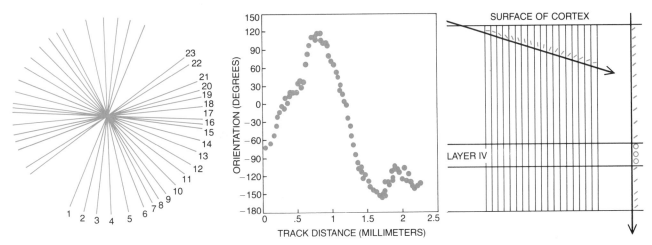

ORIENTATION PREFERENCES of 23 neurons encountered as a microelectrode penetrated the cortex obliquely are charted (*left*); the most effective tilt of the stimulus changed steadily in a counterclockwise direction. The results of a similar experiment are plotted (*center*); in this case, however, there were several reversals in direction of rotation. The results of a large number of such experiments, together with the observation that a microelectrode penetrating the cortex perpendicularly encounters only cells that prefer the same orientation (apart from the circularly symmetrical cells in layer IV, which have no preferred orientation), suggested that the cortex is subdivided into roughly parallel slabs of tissue, with each slab, called an orientation column, containing neurons with like orientation specificity (*right*).

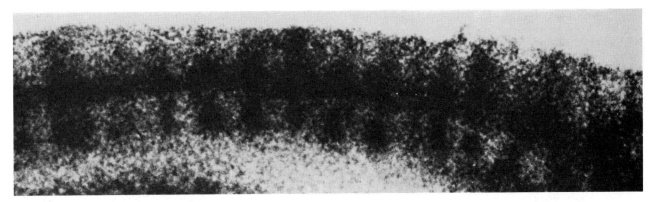

ORIENTATION COLUMNS are visualized as anatomical structures in a deoxyglucose autoradiograph made by the authors and Michael P. Stryker. Radioactively labeled deoxyglucose was injected into a monkey; it was taken up primarily by active neurons, and an early metabolite accumulated in the cells. Immediately after the injection the animal was stimulated with a pattern of vertical stripes, so that cells responding to vertical lines were most active and became most radioactive. In this section perpendicular to surface active-cell regions are narrow bands about .5 millimeter apart. Layer IV (with no orientation preference) is, as expected, uniformly radioactive.

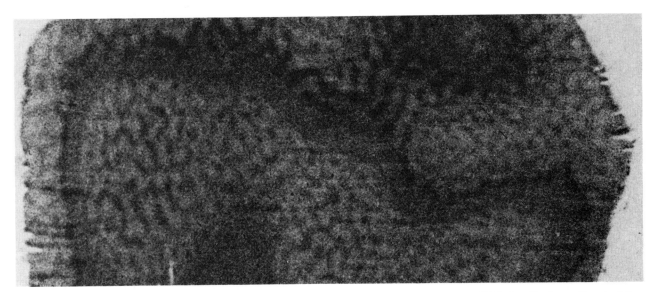

ORIENTATION PATTERN, seen face on, is unexpectedly complex. This deoxyglucose autoradiograph is of a section tangential to the somewhat curved layers of the cortex. The darker regions represent continuously labeled layer IV. In the other layers the orientation regions are intricately curved bands, something like the walls of a maze seen from above, but distance from one band to next is uniform.

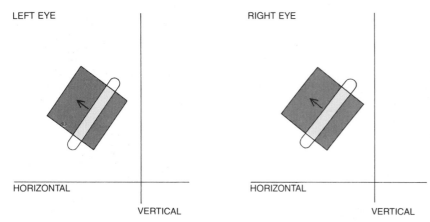

LEFT EYE   RIGHT EYE

HORIZONTAL   HORIZONTAL

VERTICAL   VERTICAL

BINOCULAR CELL in the cortex can be influenced independently by both eyes or more strongly by both eyes together. Here the left-eye and right-eye fields are mapped for a complex cell whose receptive field is in the upper left quadrant of the visual field. (The lines represent the horizontal and vertical meridians of the field, intersecting at the point of fixation.) The two receptive fields are identical, but the amount of response may differ depending on whether the left eye or the right eye is stimulated. Preference for one eye is called ocular dominance.

layers III, V and VI. The most important variation, however, is linked to eccentricity, or the distance of a cell's receptive field from the center of gaze. The size of the fields and the extent of the associated scatter in the part of the cortex that maps the center of gaze are tiny compared to the size and amount of scatter in the part that maps the far periphery. We call the pile of superimposed fields that are mapped in a penetration beginning at any point on the cortex the "aggregate field" of that point. The size of the aggregate field is obviously a function of eccentricity.

If the electrode penetrates in an oblique direction, almost parallel to the surface, the scatter in field position from cell to cell is again evident, but now there is superimposed on the scatter a consistent drift in field position, its direction dictated by the topographical map of the visual fields. And an interesting regularity is revealed: it turns out that moving the electrode about one or two millimeters always produces a displacement in visual field that is roughly enough to take one into an entirely new region. The movement in the visual field, in short, is about the same as the size of the aggregate receptive field. For the primary visual cortex this holds wherever the recording is made. At the center of gaze the fields and their associated scatter are tiny, but so is the displacement corresponding to a one-millimeter movement along the cortex. With increasing eccentricity (farther out in the visual field) both the field and scatter and the displacement become larger, in parallel fashion. It seems that every-

where a block of cortex about one or two millimeters in size is what is needed to take care of a region of the visual world equivalent to the size of an aggregate field.

These observations suggest the way the visual cortex solves a basic problem: how to analyze the visual scene in detail in the central part and much more crudely in the periphery. In the retina, which has the same problem, for obvious optical reasons the number of millimeters corresponding to a degree of visual field is constant. The retina handles the central areas in great detail by having huge numbers of ganglion cells, each subserving a tiny area of central visual field; the layer of ganglion cells in the central part of the retina is thick, whereas in the outlying parts of the retina it is very thin. The cortex, in contrast, seems to want to be uniform in thickness everywhere. Here there are none of the optical constraints imposed on the retina, and so area is simply allotted in amounts corresponding to the problem at hand.

The machinery in any square millimeter of cortex is presumably about the same as in any other. A few thousand geniculate fibers enter such a region, the cortex does its thing and perhaps 50,000 fibers leave—whether a small part of the visual world is represented in great detail or a larger part in correspondingly less detail. The uniformity of the cortex is suggested, as we indicated at the outset, by the appearance of stained sections. It is compellingly confirmed when we examine the architecture further, looking specifically at orientation and at ocular dominance.

For orientation we inquire about groupings of cells just as we did with field position, looking first at two cells sitting side by side. Two such cells almost invariably have the same optimal stimulus orientation. If the electrode is inserted in a direction perpendicular to the surface, all the cells along the path of penetration have identical or almost identical orientations (except for the cells deep in layer IV, which have no optimal orientation at all). In two perpendicular penetrations a millimeter or so apart, however, the two orientations observed are usually different. The cortex must therefore be subdivided by some kind of vertical partitioning into regions of constant receptive-field orientation. When we came on this system almost 20 years ago, it intrigued us because it fitted so well with the hierarchical schemes we had proposed to explain how complex cells are supplied by inputs from simple cells: the circuit diagrams involve connections between cells whose fields cover the same part of the visual world and that respond to the same line orientation. It seemed eminently reasonable that strongly inter-

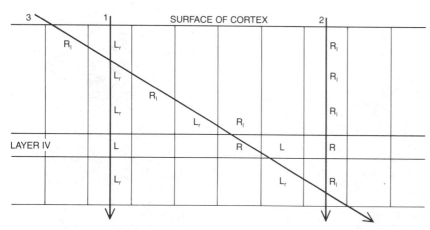

GROUPING OF CELLS according to ocular dominance was revealed by physiological studies. In one typical vertical penetration of the cortex (*1*) a microelectrode encounters only cells that respond preferentially to the left eye (L_r) and, in layer IV, cells that respond only to the left eye (*L*); in another vertical penetration (*2*) the cells all have right-eye dominance (R_l) or, in layer IV, are driven exclusively by the right eye (*R*). In an oblique penetration (*3*) there is a regular alternation of dominance by one eye or the other eye. Repeated penetrations suggest that the cortex is subdivided into regions with a cross-sectional width of about .4 millimeter and with walls perpendicular to the cortical surface and layers: the ocular-dominance columns.

connected cells should be grouped together.

If the cortex is diced up into small regions of constant receptive-field orientation, can one say anything more about the three-dimensional shape of the regions than that their walls are perpendicular to the surface? Are neighboring regions related in any systematic way or are regions subserving all the possible orientations scattered over the cortex at random? We began to study these questions simply by penetrating the cortex obliquely or parallel to the surface. When we first did this experiment in about 1961, the result was so surprising that we could hardly believe it. Instead of a random assortment of successive orientations there was an amazing orderliness. Each time the electrode moved forward as little as 25 or 50 micrometers (thousandths of a millimeter) the optimal orientation changed by a small step, about 10 degrees on the average; the steps continued in the same direction, clockwise or counterclockwise, through a total angle of anywhere from 90 to 270 degrees. Occasionally such a sequence would reverse direction suddenly, from a clockwise progression to a counterclockwise one or vice versa. These reversals were unpredictable, usually coming after steady progressions of from 90 to 270 degrees.

Since making this first observation we have seen similar order in almost every monkey. Either there is a steady progression in orientation or, less frequently, there are stretches in which orientation stays constant. The successive changes in orientation are small enough so that it is hard to be sure that the regions of constant orientation are finite in size; it could be that the optimal orientation changes in some sense continuously as the electrode moves along the cortex.

We became increasingly interested in the three-dimensional shape of these regional subdivisions. From considerations of geometry alone the existence of small or zero changes in every direction during a horizontal or tangential penetration points to parallel slabs of tissue containing cells with like orientation specificity, with each slab perpendicular to the surface. The slabs would not necessarily be planar, like slices of bread; seen from above they might well have the form of swirls, which could easily explain the reversals in the direction of orientation changes. Recording large numbers of cells in several parallel electrode penetrations seemed to confirm this prediction, but it was hard to examine more than a tiny region of brain with the microelectrode.

Fortunately an ideal anatomical method was invented at just the right time for us. This was the 2-deoxyglucose technique for assessing brain activity, devised by Louis Sokoloff and his group at the National Institute of Mental Health [see "The Chemistry of the Brain," by Leslie L. Iversen; SCIENTIFIC AMERICAN Offprint 1440]. The method capitalizes on the fact that brain cells depend mainly on glucose as a source of metabolic energy and that the closely similar compound 2-deoxyglucose can to some extent masquerade as glucose. If deoxyglucose is injected into an animal, it is taken up actively by neurons as though it were glucose; the more active the neuron, the greater the uptake. The compound begins to be metabolized, but for reasons best known to biochemists the sequence stops with a metabolite that cannot cross the cell wall and therefore accumulates within the cell.

The Sokoloff procedure is to inject an animal with deoxyglucose that has been labeled with the radioactive isotope carbon 14, stimulate the animal in a way calculated to activate certain neurons

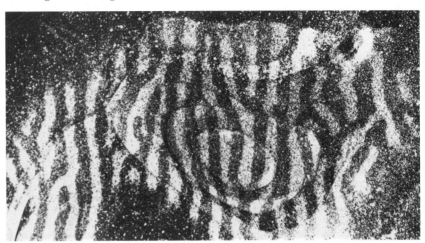

ANATOMICAL CONFIRMATION of ocular-dominance columns came from various staining methods and from axonal-transport autoradiographs such as those shown in color on page 41. This composite autoradiograph visualizing the pattern over an area some 10 millimeters wide was made by cutting out and pasting together the regions representing layer IV in a number of parallel sections; the one in bottom illustration on page 41 and others at different depths.

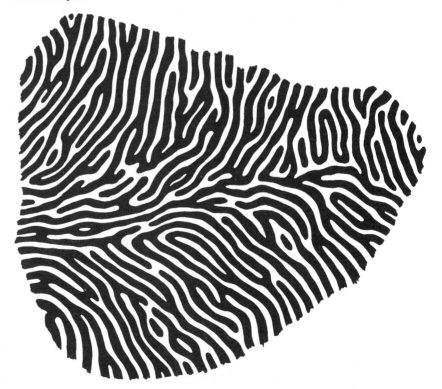

RECONSTRUCTION of the ocular-dominance pattern over the entire exposed part of the right primary visual cortex was made by the authors and Simon LeVay from a series of sections stained by a reduced-silver method he developed. The left-hand margin is at the medial edge of occipital lobe, where cortex folds downward; pattern is enlarged about six diameters.

and then immediately examine the brain for radioactivity, which reveals active areas where cells will have taken up more deoxyglucose than those in quiescent areas. The usual way of examining the brain for this purpose is to cut very thin slices of it (as one would for microscopic examination) and press them against a photographic plate sensitive to the radioactive particles. When the film is developed, any areas that were in contact with radioactive material are seen as dark masses of developed silver grains. Together with Michael P. Stryker we adapted the Sokoloff method to our problem, injecting an anesthetized animal with deoxyglucose and then moving a pattern of black and white vertical stripes back and forth 1.5 meters in front of the animal for 45 minutes. We then cut the brain into slices, either perpendicular to the surface of the cortex or parallel to it.

The autoradiographs quickly confirmed the physiological results. Sections cut perpendicular to the surface showed narrow bands of radioactivity about every 570 micrometers (roughly half a millimeter), extending through the full thickness of the cortex. Evidently these were the regions containing cells responsive to vertical lines. The deep

part of layer IV was uniformly radioactive, as was expected from the fact that the cells in the layer have circularly symmetrical receptive fields and show no orientation selectivity.

Sections cut parallel to the surface showed an unexpectedly complex set of periodically spaced bands, often swirling, frequently branching and rejoining, only here and there forming regular parallel slabs. What was particularly striking was the uniformity of the distance from one band to the next over the entire cortex. This fitted perfectly with the idea of a uniform cortex. Moreover, the distance between stripes fitted well with the idea that the cortical machinery must repeat itself at least every millimeter. If the distance were, for example, 10 millimeters from vertical through 180 degrees and back to vertical, sizable parts of the visual field would lack cells sensitive to any given orientation, making for a sketchy and extremely bizarre representation of the visual scene.

The final variable whose associated architecture needs to be considered is eye preference. In microelectrode studies neighboring cells proved almost invariably to prefer the same eye. If in vertical penetrations the first cell we en-

countered preferred the right eye, then so did all the cells, right down to the bottom of layer VI; if the first cell preferred the left eye, so did all the rest. Any penetration favored one eye or the other with equal probability. (Since the cells of layer IV are monocular, there it was a matter not of eye preference but of eye monopoly.) If the penetration was oblique or horizontal, there was an alternation of left and right preferences, with a rather abrupt switchover about every half millimeter. The cortex thus proved to be diced up into a second set of regions separated by vertical walls that extend through the full cortical thickness. The ocular-dominance system was apparently quite independent of the orientation system, because in oblique or tangential penetrations the two sequences had no apparent relation to each other.

The basis of these ocular-dominance columns, as they have come to be called, seems to be quite simple. The terminals of geniculate fibers, some subserving the left eye and others the right, group themselves as they enter the cortex so that in layer IV there is no mixing. This produces left-eye and right-eye patches at roughly half-millimeter intervals. A neuron above or below layer IV receives connections from that layer from up to about a millimeter away in every direction. Probably the strongest connections are from the region of layer IV closest to the neuron, so that it is presumably dominated by whichever eye feeds that region.

Again we were most curious to learn what these left-eye and right-eye regions might look like in three dimensions; any of several geometries could lead to the cross-sectional appearance the physiology had suggested. The answer first came from studies with the silver-degeneration method for mapping connections, devised by Walle J. H. Nauta of the Massachusetts Institute of Technology. Since then we have found three other independent anatomical methods for demonstrating these columns.

A particularly effective method (because it enables one to observe in a single animal the arrangement of columns over the entire primary visual cortex) is based on the phenomenon of axonal transport. The procedure is to inject a radioactively labeled amino acid into an area of nervous tissue. A cell body takes up the amino acid, presumably incorporates it into a protein and then transports it along the axon to its terminals. When we injected the material into one eye of a monkey, the retinal ganglion cells took it up and transported it along their axons, the optic-nerve fibers. We could then examine the destinations of these fibers in the lateral geniculate nuclei by coating tissue slices with a silver emulsion and developing the emulsion; the radioactive label showed up clearly in

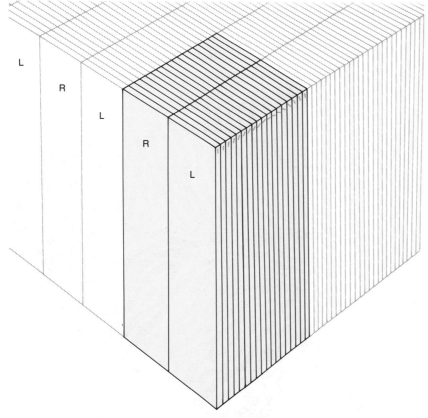

BLOCK OF CORTEX about a millimeter square and two millimeters deep (*light color*) can be considered an elementary unit of the primary visual cortex. It contains one set of orientation slabs subserving all orientations and one set of ocular-dominance slabs subserving both eyes. The pattern is reiterated throughout the primary visual area. The placing of the boundaries (at the right or the left eye, at a vertical, horizontal or oblique orientation) is arbitrary; representation of the slabs as flat planes intersecting at right angles is an oversimplification.

the three complementary layers of the geniculate on each side.

This method does not ordinarily trace a path from one axon terminal across a synapse to the next neuron and its terminals, however, and we wanted to follow the path all the way to the cortex. In 1971 Bernice Grafstein of the Cornell University Medical College discovered that after a large enough injection in the eye of a mouse some of the radioactive material escaped from the optic-nerve terminals and was taken up by the cells in the geniculate and transported along their axons to the cortex. We had the thought that a similarly large injection in a monkey, combined with autoradiography, might demonstrate the geniculate terminals from one eye in layer IV of the visual cortex.

Our first attempt yielded dismayingly negative results, with only faint hints of a few silver grains visible in layer IV. It was only after several weeks that we realized that by resorting to dark-field microscopy we could take advantage of the light-scattering properties of silver grains and so increase the sensitivity of the method. We borrowed a dark-field condenser, and when we looked at our first slide under the microscope, there shining in all their glory were the periodic patches of label in layer IV [see top illustration on page 41].

The next step was to try to see the pattern face on by sectioning the cortex parallel to its surface. The monkey cortex is dome-shaped, and so a section parallel to the surface and tangent to layer IV shows that layer as a circle or an oval, while a section below layer IV shows it as a ring. By assembling a series of such ovals and rings from a set of sections one can reconstruct the pattern over a wide expanse of cortex.

From the reconstructions it was immediately obvious that the main overall pattern is one of parallel stripes representing terminals belonging to the injected eye, separated by gaps representing the other eye. The striping pattern is not regular like wallpaper. (We remind ourselves occasionally that this is, after all, biology!) Here and there a stripe representing one eye branches into two stripes, or else it ends blindly at a point where a stripe from the other eye branches. The irregularities are commonest near the center of gaze and along the line that maps the horizon. The stripes always seem to be perpendicular to the border between the primary visual cortex and its neighbor, area 18, and here the regularity is greatest. Such general rules seem to apply to all macaque brains, although the details of the pattern vary from one individual to the next and even from one hemisphere to the other in the same monkey.

The width of a set of two stripes is constant, about .8 millimeter, over the

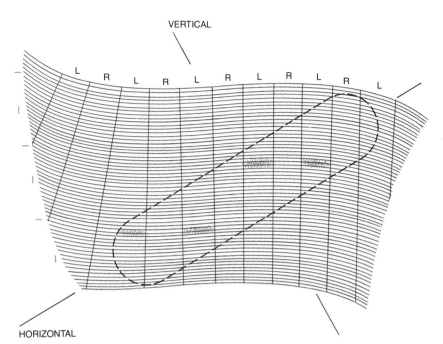

entire primary visual cortex, once more emphasizing the uniformity of the cortex. Again the widths fit perfectly with the idea that all of the apparatus needed to look after an area the size of an aggregate field must be contained within any square millimeter of cortex. The two techniques, deoxyglucose labeling and amino acid transport, have the great advantage of being mutually compatible, so that we have been able to apply both together, one to mark orientation lines and the other to see the ocular-dominance columns. The number of brains examined so far is too small to justify any final conclusions, but the two systems appear to be quite independent, neither parallel nor at right angles but intersecting at random.

The function served by ocular-dominance columns is still a mystery. We know there are neurons with all grades of eye preference throughout the entire binocular part of the visual fields, and it may be that a regular, patterned system of converging inputs guarantees that the distribution will be uniform, with neither eye favored by accident in any one place. Why there should be all these grades of eye preference everywhere is itself not clear, but our guess is that it has something to do with stereoscopic depth perception.

Given what has been learned about the primary visual cortex, it is clear that one can consider an elementary piece of cortex to be a block about a millimeter square and two millimeters deep. To know the organization of this chunk of tissue is to know the organization for all of area 17; the whole must be mainly an iterated version of this elementary unit. Of course the elementary unit should not be thought of as a discrete, separable block. Whether the set of orientation slabs begins with a slab representing a vertical orientation, an oblique one or a horizontal one is completely arbitrary; so too is whether an ocular-dominance sequence begins with a left-plus-right pair of dominance slabs or a right-plus-left pair. The same thing is true for a unit crystal of sodium chloride or for any complex repetitive pattern such as is found in wallpaper.

What, then, does the visual scene really look like as it is projected onto the visual cortex? Suppose an animal fixes its gaze on some point and the only object in the visual field is a straight line above and a bit to the left of the point where the gaze is riveted. If each active cell were to light up, and if one could stand above the cortex and look down at it, what would the pattern be? To make the problem more interesting, suppose the pattern is seen by one eye only. In view of the architecture just described the pattern turns out to be not a line but merely a set of regularly spaced patches [see illustration above]. The reasoning can be checked directly by exposing a monkey with one eye closed to a set of vertical stripes and making a deoxyglucose autoradiograph. The resulting pattern should not be a great surprise: it is a set of regularly spaced patches, which simply represents the intersection of the two sets of column systems. Imagine the surprise and bewilderment of a little green man looking at such a version of the outside world!

Why evolution has gone to the trouble of designing such an elaborate architecture is a question that continues to fascinate us. Perhaps the most plausible notion is that the column systems are a solution to the problem of portraying more than two dimensions on a two-dimensional surface. The cortex is dealing with at least four sets of values: two for the x and y position variables in the visual field, one for orientation and one for the different degrees of eye preference. The two surface coordinates are used up in designating field position; the other two variables are accommodated by dicing up the cortex with subdivisions so fine that one can run through a complete set of orientations or eye preferences and meanwhile have a shift in visual-field position that is small with respect to the resolution in that part of the visual world.

The strategy of subdividing the cortex with small vertical partitions is certainly not limited to the primary visual area. Such subdivisions were first seen in the somatic sensory area by Vernon B. Mountcastle of the Johns Hopkins University School of Medicine about 10 years before our work in the visual area. In the somatic sensory area, as we pointed out above, the basic topography is a map of the opposite half of the body, but superimposed on that there is a twofold system of subdivisions, with some areas where neurons respond to the movement of the joints or pressure on the skin and other areas where they respond to touch or the bending of hairs. As in the case of the visual columns, a complete set here (one area for each kind of neuron) occupies a distance of about a millimeter. These subdivisions are analogous to ocular-dominance columns in that they are determined in the first instance by inputs to the cortex (from either the left or the right eye and from either deep receptors or receptors in the upper skin layers) rather than by connections within the cortex, such as those that determine orientation selectivity and the associated system of orientation regions.

The columnar subdivisions associated with the visual and somatic sensory systems are the best-understood ones, but there are indications of similar vertical subdivisions in some other areas: several higher visual areas, sensory parietal regions recently studied by Mountcastle and the auditory region, where Thomas J. Imig, H. O. Adrián and John F. Brugge of the University of Wisconsin Medical School and their colleagues have found subdivisions in which the two ears seem alternately to add their information or to compete.

For most of these physiologically defined systems (except the visual ones) there are so far no anatomical correlates. On the other hand, in the past few years several anatomists, notably Edward G. Jones of the Washington University School of Medicine and Nauta and Patricia Goldman at M.I.T., have shown that connections from one region of the cortex to another (for example from the somatic sensory area on one side to the corresponding area on the other side) terminate in patches that have a regular periodicity of about a millimeter. Here the columns are evident morphologically, but one has no idea of the physiological interpretation. It is clear, however, that fine periodic subdivisions are a very general feature of the cerebral cortex. Indeed, Mountcastle's original observation of that feature may be said to supply a fourth profound insight into cortical organization.

It would surely be wrong to assume that this account of the visual cortex in any way exhausts the subject. Color, movement and stereoscopic depth are probably all dealt with in the cortex, but to what extent or how is still not clear. There are indications from work we and others have done on depth and from work on color by Semir Zeki of University College London that higher cortical visual areas to which the primary area projects directly or indirectly may be specialized to handle these variables, but we are a long way from knowing what the handling involves.

What happens beyond the primary visual area, and how is the information on orientation exploited at later stages? Is one to imagine ultimately finding a cell that responds specifically to some very particular item? (Usually one's grandmother is selected as the particular item, for reasons that escape us.) Our answer is that we doubt there is such a cell, but we have no good alternative to offer. To speculate broadly on how the brain may work is fortunately not the only course open to investigators. To explore the brain is more fun and seems to be more profitable.

There was a time, not so long ago, when one looked at the millions of neurons in the various layers of the cortex and wondered if anyone would ever have any idea of their function. Did they all work in parallel, like the cells of the liver or the kidney, achieving their objectives by pure bulk, or were they each doing something special? For the visual cortex the answer seems now to be known in broad outline: Particular stimuli turn neurons on or off; groups of neurons do indeed perform particular transformations. It seems reasonable to think that if the secrets of a few regions such as this one can be unlocked, other regions will also in time give up their secrets.

ACTUAL PATTERN of cortical activity was elicited by exposing only the left eye to a set of vertical stripes. The deoxyglucose autoradiograph is of a tangential section in the outer layers of the cortex. The pattern of regularly spaced dark patches of radioactivity represents intersection of ocular-dominance and orientation systems. Magnification is about eight diameters.

5

Negative Aftereffects in Visual Perception

by Olga Eizner Favreau and Michael C. Corballis
December 1976

You will see one if you stare at a waterfall for a short time and then look away; the surrounding scene will seem to move slowly upward. The study of such illusions yields information on perceptual systems

It is a common experience to look at a bright light and to find that a dark image of the object remains in the visual field for some time afterward. The phenomenon is called a negative afterimage (negative because the object was bright and the image is dark). A similar phenomenon can be experienced by staring for several minutes at something that is moving in a uniform direction, as a waterfall does, and then turning the gaze away; the surrounding scene will appear to drift slowly in the opposite direction. This is a negative aftereffect. Afterimages and aftereffects are illusions, reminding one that the senses are sometimes imperfect mediators between the external world and one's perception of it. The study of such illusions is valuable in psychology for the clues they provide to how the sense organs and the nervous system function in processing information.

Afterimages and aftereffects are encountered in a variety of forms. For example, afterimages of colored objects appear in colors that are complementary to the colors of the objects. If you stare at a patch of green for a minute or so and then look at a blank field, you can expect to see a reddish patch of the same shape [see illustration on page 54].

In addition to motion aftereffects of the kind evoked by watching a waterfall one can experience figural aftereffects. For example, if you look at a line that is tilted about 15 degrees from the vertical, a line that is actually vertical may appear to be tilted in the opposite direction [see bottom illustration on page 58]. A related aftereffect can be observed if you look at a curved line for a time; a straight line then seems to curve the other way.

Aftereffects are by no means limited to vision. If someone is blindfolded and then runs a finger back and forth along a curved rod, a straight rod will seem to be curved the other way. Similarly, as has been demonstrated by Stuart M. Anstis of York University, if one listens repeatedly to a tone that increases in intensity, a tone of constant intensity is likely to sound as though it is decreasing in intensity. Here we shall focus on visual aftereffects, since they have been the most intensively examined.

A number of investigators in the 19th century thought motion aftereffects might be related to movements of the eyes. Exposure to a moving pattern induces the eyes to follow the motion of the pattern. If the eyes tend to persist in the same pattern of scanning when the movement is no longer there, a stationary pattern might then seem to move in the opposite direction.

In 1850, however, this hypothesis was discredited by the Belgian physicist Joseph Plateau on the basis of work with rotating spirals. Such a spiral appears either to expand or to contract, depending on the direction of rotation. Plateau found that if one watches an expanding spiral for a few minutes, a stationary spiral then seems to contract; conversely, a contracting spiral induces an aftereffect of expansion. The spiral aftereffect cannot be explained simply in terms of eye movements, because both expansion and contraction consist of movement in all directions at once.

Another explanation for aftereffects is the concept of normalization proposed by J. J. Gibson of Cornell University. He argued that a prolonged exposure to a stimulus that deviates in some way from an established norm might serve to redefine the norm. For example, an exposure to a line that is tilted slightly from the vertical might induce the observer to recalibrate his conception of the vertical toward the line. A truly vertical line would then be seen as being tilted in the other direction. This hypothesis may be partly correct, but it cannot easily account for aftereffects

that arise when no obvious norm is involved. As Donald E. Mitchell and Darwin W. Muir of Dalhousie University have shown, the tilt aftereffect induced with a stimulus of oblique lines is similar in both magnitude and direction to the aftereffects induced with vertical and horizontal lines.

In recent years attempts to understand visual aftereffects have drawn increasingly on concepts derived from the growing body of knowledge of the neurophysiology of the visual system. Although most of this work is based on recordings made with microelectrodes from individual neurons, or nerve cells, in the visual system of such animals as cats and monkeys, a number of psychologists have been quick to extrapolate the findings to human vision. The exchange has also gone the other way: concepts derived from work on aftereffects in human beings preceded fundamental discoveries in the neurophysiology of vision in other primates. We hope to convey something of the flavor of this exchange between disciplines.

Light reaching the eye is focused by the lens to form a two-dimensional image on the retina. Light-sensitive receptors there convert the image into a spatial pattern of neural impulses. The impulses are transmitted from the receptors to a layer of neurons called bipolar cells and then to another layer called retinal ganglion cells. Fibers from the retinal ganglion cells make up the optic nerve, which carries the neural information from the retina to the brain.

Negative and complementary afterimages probably depend largely on the properties of cells in the retina. It is easy to demonstrate that an afterimage moves about as one moves one's eyes and that its location is perfectly correlated with the position of the eyes; it is as though the afterimage were painted on the retina. In contrast, objects actually present in the visual field appear to remain fixed if one moves one's eyes. These observations hold only for normal, voluntary eye movements. The situation is reversed if one moves an eye passively, as by pressing at the corner of the eye with a finger; then objects in the real world appear to move but an afterimage remains motionless. Both kinds of observation show that afterimages are formed at a level of processing preceding the one where the perceived location of objects in space is "corrected" for voluntary eye movements.

It is also easy to show that afterimages do not transfer from one eye to the other. The reader can verify this finding by looking at the illustration at the right for about 40 seconds with a hand over one eye. The afterimage will then be visible against a plain surface only to the exposed eye.

One can explain these phenomena by supposing cells in the retina, including the receptors, become temporarily fatigued or adapted after a long stimulation. According to this reasoning, if one looks at, say, a white patch, cells responsive to white light become less responsive, leaving an impression of a dark patch if the gaze is shifted to a uniform field. Complementary afterimages (red following green, for example) can be explained in a similar way.

Neurons beyond the receptors may also contribute to afterimages. They include the bipolar and ganglion cells in the retina and possibly cells in the lateral geniculate nucleus, a relay station in the brain that receives its input directly from the retinal ganglion cells. Among the retinal ganglion cells and the lateral geniculate cells are cells that typically exhibit what is termed "opponent process" organization, meaning that a cell increases its normal rate of firing in response to one color but decreases it in response to the complementary color. Opponent-process cells might contribute to afterimages in two ways. Suppose one views a uniform green field for a period of time. The cells that fire at an increased rate for green (they are called green-on, red-off cells) may become fatigued, so that if one subsequently views a uniform white field, the reduced firing of these cells is interpreted as redness. Conversely, red-on, green-off cells would be depressed while one was looking at a green field and might subsequently "rebound" to enhance the impression of redness.

Whereas afterimages depend on the fatigue of cells in the early stages of visual processing, figural and motion aftereffects appear to depend on properties of neurons at a higher level, perhaps in the visual cortex. The study of such aftereffects was greatly stimulated by the pioneering discoveries of David H. Hubel and Torsten N. Wiesel of the

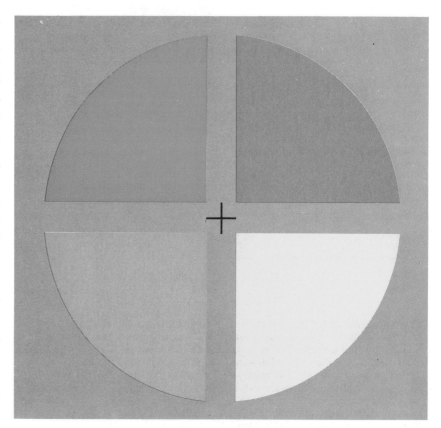

NEGATIVE AFTERIMAGE is the simplest kind of negative aftereffect. Here the afterimage will appear in the color that is complementary to the color you look at. If you fix your gaze on the cross at the center of the colors for about a minute and then look at the gray field at the bottom of the page, you should see patches that are in the complementary colors of the original: the green, yellow, blue and red will be replaced respectively by red, blue, yellow and green.

Harvard Medical School on the properties of neurons in the visual cortex of the cat brain [see "The Visual Cortex of the Brain," by David H. Hubel; SCIENTIFIC AMERICAN, Offprint 168]. Hubel and Wiesel found cells that they classified hierarchically as simple, complex and hypercomplex. Simple cells respond to edges, slits or lines. The edge, slit or line must be precisely located and oriented in the visual field to cause a given cell to fire at the maximum rate. Although location is not so critical for complex and hypercomplex cells, they have the added characteristic of responding maximally when the preferred stimulus is in motion in a direction perpendicular to its orientation. Many of these cells are also directionally selective in that they respond to motion in one direction but not to motion in the opposite direction.

In 1961, two years after the first report by Hubel and Wiesel, N. Stuart Sutherland, who is now at the University of Sussex, suggested that cortical cells of the kind described by the Harvard workers might underlie aftereffects of motion and orientation. His explanation, like the one we have described for afterimages, invoked the concept of neural fatigue. According to Sutherland, the perception of the orientation of a line would involve a kind of averaging of the activity of all the line detectors that respond to the line. If one looks at, say, a vertical line, the neurons most sensitive to verticalness are the most active and there is no overall bias due to the activity of cells sensitive to other orientations. The decision about the orientation of the line therefore corresponds to reality.

Now suppose the observer looks for some time at a line that is tilted 15 degrees clockwise. Line detectors maximally sensitive to the 15-degree line become fatigued, so that when the observer looks at the vertical line, the balance of activity is shifted counterclockwise away from the vertical. A similar process could underlie motion aftereffects.

The recognition that single cells in the cat's brain are simultaneously sensitive to more than one specific feature of environmental stimuli, such as orientation and brightness, introduced the possibility of discovering aftereffects with multiple components. The possibility was first realized by Celeste McCollough of Oberlin College. She reasoned that human beings probably have line detectors similar to the ones found in cats and that since people, unlike cats, also have color vision it might not be unreasonable to suppose that human line detectors are specialized for color as well as for orientation. If they are, one might be able to demonstrate aftereffects that depend on both the orientation and the color of lines.

McCollough accomplished the dem-

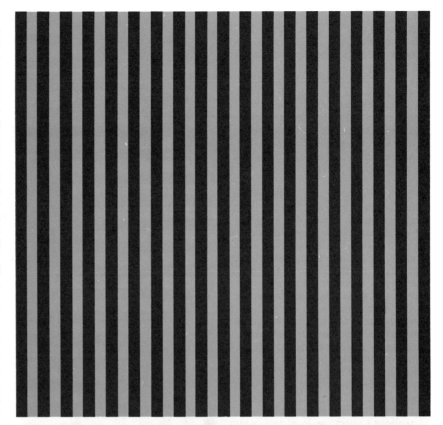

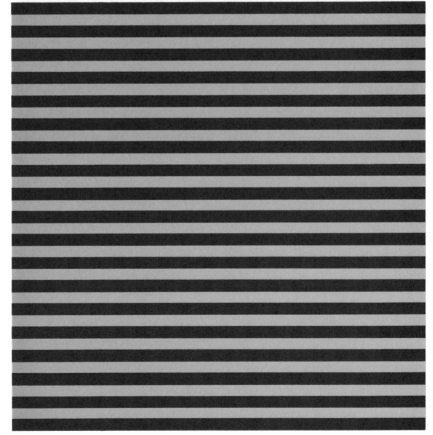

CONTINGENT AFTEREFFECT is demonstrated by these two grids and the pattern in the illustration on page 56. Look alternately at one grid and then the other for about 10 seconds each for 10 minutes. Then look at the pattern on page 56. Its horizontal lines should appear reddish and its vertical lines greenish. If the page is turned 90 degrees, the color relations reverse. The phenomenon is termed an orientation-contingent color aftereffect.

onstration in the following way. Subjects looked at grids of horizontal blue and black lines alternating every few seconds with grids of vertical orange and black lines. After about 10 minutes they were shown grids of horizontal and of vertical white and black lines. The horizontal grids appeared to have a faint orange color and the vertical grids were tinged with blue. This result can be described as an orientation-contingent color aftereffect; it is generally known as the McCollough effect.

It is unlikely that the McCollough effect is retinal in origin. For one thing it is clear that the perceived colors are not simply complementary afterimages, since either color can be seen in the same retinal location, depending only on the orientation of the lines in the grid. Moreover, it is not necessary to gaze fixedly at the figures in order to get the McCollough effect.

Another aspect of the McCollough effect that differentiates it from simple afterimages is its extreme persistence. With an adaptation period of 10 or 15 minutes the effect may still be visible days or even weeks later. Because of these properties it is generally believed that the mechanisms responsible for the McCollough effect are localized in the visual cortex of the cerebrum. Three years after McCollough's discovery Hubel and Wiesel reported that the visual cortex of the monkey does in fact contain neurons sensitive to both the orientation and the color of a stimulus.

Other reports of contingent aftereffects have followed McCollough's work. Norva Hepler of McGill University and Charles F. Stromeyer and R. J. W. Mansfield of Harvard University independently discovered that color aftereffects can be made contingent on the direction of motion of a pattern. For example, if an observer alternately watches a spiral rotating clockwise in green light and counterclockwise in red light, a black-and-white spiral may subsequently appear pinkish if it is rotated clockwise and greenish if it is rotated counterclockwise.

We and Victor F. Emerson, working at McGill, discovered that it is possible to induce the converse of this contingency. (The finding was also reported by Anstis and John E. W. Mayhew.) After watching a green clockwise spiral alternating with a red counterclockwise spiral observers report that a stationary spiral appears to move briefly counterclockwise when it is green and clockwise when it is red. This is a color-contingent motion aftereffect. Like the motion-contingent color aftereffect, it is long-lasting, that is, although it is brief for any one exposure to a colored spiral, it can reappear when the spiral is looked at again. Both the color-contingent motion aftereffect and the motion-contingent

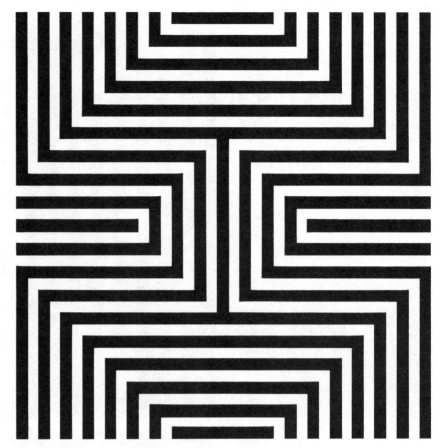

BLACK-AND-WHITE PATTERN, viewed in conjunction with grids on page 55, produces the orientation-contingent color aftereffect. Such multiple-component aftereffects are called McCollough effects after Celeste McCollough of Oberlin Colege, who discovered them.

color aftereffect can reappear if an observer is shown the test patterns 24 hours after adaptation.

The evidence we have reviewed so far seems to support the view that aftereffects depend on the properties of feature detectors that bear a close functional resemblance to the neurons described by Hubel and Wiesel. Nevertheless, investigators in both neurophysiology and human perception have recently sought to prove the existence of detectors that respond to more integrated properties of the visual display. Indeed, some workers now believe the neurons studied by Hubel and Wiesel do not function simply as edge, slit or line detectors but also contribute to an analysis of the spatial frequencies (the spacing of more or less regularly repeating elements) in the total display. It has been found that individual neurons in the visual cortex of the cat respond selectively to sinusoidal gratings (parallel bars having a brightness that varies in a sinusoidal manner across the grating) only within a narrow range of spatial frequencies [see "Contrast and Spatial Frequency," by Fergus W. Campbell and Lamberto Maffei; SCIENTIFIC AMERICAN Offprint 1308].

A number of aftereffects can be attributed to detectors of spatial frequency. For example, Colin Blakemore and

Peter Sutton of the University of Cambridge discovered that if one looks at a striped pattern for some minutes and then views a grating with the same orientation but slightly narrower bars, the bars seem even narrower and more closely spaced than they really are. Conversely, broader bars seem broader [see bottom illustration on page 59].

The explanation proposed by Blakemore and Sutton was similar to the one advanced by Sutherland to explain tilt and motion aftereffects. They suggested that a grating of a particular frequency arouses activity in a subpopulation of frequency-detecting neurons. The distribution of activity is averaged to provide a perceptual impression of what the displayed frequency is. Preadaptation to some other spatial frequency would have depressed the activity of neurons sensitive to that frequency and so would skew the distribution away from the distribution normally evoked by the displayed pattern.

Color aftereffects can also be made contingent on spatial frequency. W. J. Lovegrove and Ray F. Over of the University of Queensland had subjects watch a vertical grating of one spatial frequency in red light alternating with a vertical grating of a different spatial frequency in green light. Afterward a black-and-white test grating of the first frequency appeared greenish and a grating of the second frequency appeared pinkish. Color aftereffects occurred, however, only if the frequency of one grating was at least twice that of the other and if the frequency of at least one grating was higher than three cycles per degree of visual angle. Lovegrove and Over suggested that their results could be explained in terms of the adaptation of neural units tuned for both color and spatial frequency.

A useful way to check on the location in the visual system of the neurons responsible for aftereffects is to test for interactions of the eyes. For example, one can induce an aftereffect in one eye and then ask whether the observer sees it when he looks with the other eye. Neurons in the visual pathway from the retina to the visual cortex are driven by one eye up to and including the lateral geniculate nucleus. In the visual cortex some neurons are driven monocularly (by an input to one eye only) and others are driven binocularly (by an input to either eye). Most of the cells in the superior colliculus (another part of the visual-processing system) are driven binocularly. Hence if an aftereffect is observed to transfer from one eye to the other, one can infer that it is mediated by cells in either the visual cortex or the superior colliculus. Since neurons in the superior colliculus appear to be sensitive mainly to motion, however, their role (if they have one) would be confined to motion aftereffects.

It has generally been found that figural and motion aftereffects, unlike afterimages, do transfer from one eye to the other, although their strength is reduced in the process. These aftereffects are therefore probably mediated by both monocularly and binocularly driven neurons. In the eye that was exposed to the adapting pattern both kinds of neurons would mediate the effect. In the other eye, however, only the neurons driven binocularly would be involved, which accounts for the reduction in strength.

Contingent aftereffects where one of the components is color apparently do not transfer from one eye to the other. This finding suggested that they may be mediated by monocularly driven neurons. Some evidence indicates, however, that this hypothesis may not be altogether correct. Experiments conducted by T. R. Vidyasagar of the University of Manchester have indicated that orientation-contingent color aftereffects can involve neurons that require an input to both eyes. Such neurons are binocular, but they could not mediate an interocular transfer. It seems possible that other contingent aftereffects may also involve binocular neurons of this type.

Gerald M. Murch of Portland State

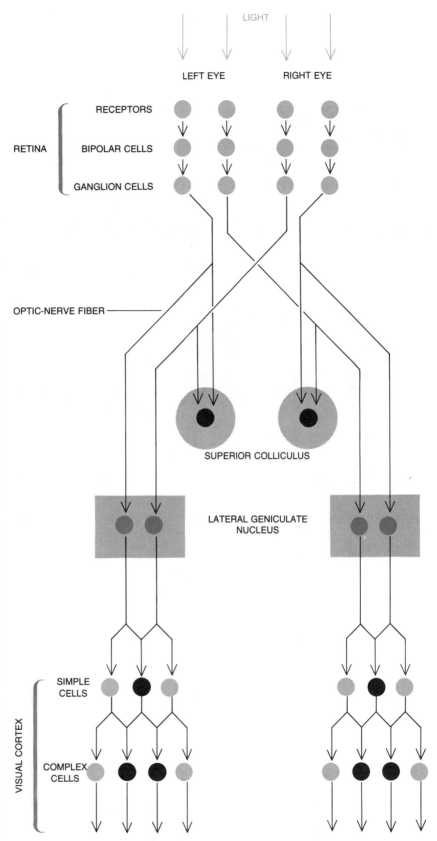

VISUAL SYSTEM is depicted schematically to show the flow of information. The neurons, or nerve cells, represented in color are driven by only one eye, whereas the ones shown in black are driven by both eyes. Hence if an aftereffect that has been induced in one eye is observed to transfer to the other eye, one can infer that it is mediated by cells either in the visual cortex of the brain or in the superior colliculus. Afterimages, in contrast to aftereffects, do not transfer from one eye to the other, so that they evidently originate in early stages of visual processing.

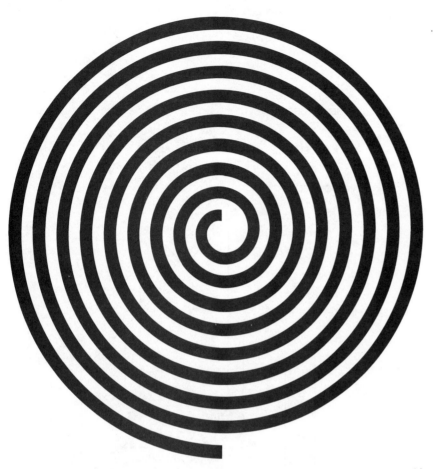

SPIRAL AFTEREFFECT is caused by putting a spiral on a turntable and rotating it at 33⅓ revolutions per minute. When the spiral is stopped, it seems to move in the other direction.

University has demonstrated that the color and motion components of an aftereffect can be dissociated. He has also shown that the motion component transfers from one eye to the other and the color component does not. Murch's procedure involved an adaptation phase and a test phase. In the adaptation phase he presented to the right eye a spiral whose motion was alternated between clockwise and counterclockwise, and at the same time he presented to the left eye the contingent color, alternately red and green. In the test phase the observer looked at stationary red or green spirals with first one eye and then the other. The contingent aftereffect (clockwise movement of the green spiral and counterclockwise movement of the red one) was reported only when the observer used his left eye. The adaptation to motion thus transferred from one eye to the other but the information about the contingent colors did not.

Murch's elegant experiment raises a general question about the nature of contingent aftereffects. Until recently it had been widely assumed that they are due solely to the adaptation of "multiple duty" neurons tuned to the different components, such as color and orientation, that underlie the aftereffects. Murch and other workers have questioned this assumption, suggesting instead that the contingency may depend on associative connections between different classes of neurons, each type tuned to a single component of the visual experience. Although Murch's experiment does not rule out the participation of multiple-duty neurons in the mediation of contingent aftereffects, it does introduce the possibility that such aftereffects can also be mediated by associations among previously independent neurons.

The possibility that contingent aftereffects may depend on the formation of associative connections rather than (or perhaps in addition to) fatigue has been suggested for another reason, namely the persistence of many contingent aftereffects. As we have mentioned, they can be detected days or even weeks after the adaptation period. We know of no neurophysiological evidence that fatigue or the adaptation of single neurons ever persists for such a long time.

Indeed, the persistence may not be confined to contingent aftereffects, although the question of whether or not an aftereffect is contingent is sometimes a fine point. Richard F. Masland of McGill showed that features of the spiral aftereffect can persist for as long as 24 hours. One of us (Favreau) has found that it may still be present a week later. The decrease in magnitude of the spiral aftereffect is rapid during the first few minutes, but thereafter the rate of decrease is markedly slower. For this reason Masland suggested that the aftereffect has two components: a rapidly decaying component directly due to the adaptation of motion detectors and a more slowly decaying, more persistent component caused by the conditioned adaptation of the detectors. In conditioned adaptation, although the motion detectors would not remain fatigued for the entire period during which the aftereffect persists, the spiral configuration, having become associated with fatigue, could cause the detectors to return to a state resembling fatigue.

Although the concept of conditioned adaptation or fatigue could be useful in explaining the long-term persistence of negative aftereffects, it presents a stumbling block. If the various attributes of the inducing stimulus, such as spiral configuration and clockwise motion, become associated with one another, one would expect to obtain positive aftereffects rather than negative ones. Thus, for example, a stationary spiral would

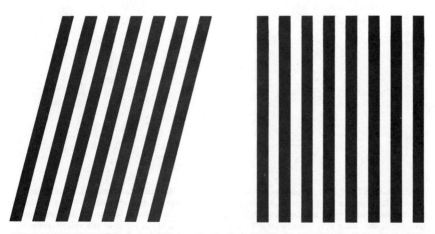

TILT AFTEREFFECT appears when one has looked steadily for about five minutes at the tilted lines. Thereafter lines that are actually vertical will seem to tilt in the opposite direction.

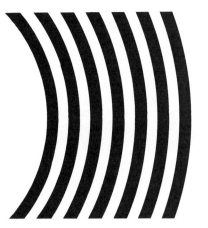

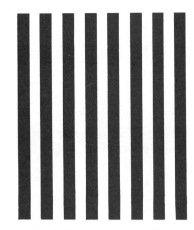

CURVE AFTEREFFECT results from looking at curved lines for 10 minutes, moving the eyes only along the central portion. The straight lines will then appear to curve the opposite way.

If contingent aftereffects do depend on the formation of associative connections between visual units, the question arises of how such connections are established. One possibility is that information from different sets of feature-extracting neurons converges in a mutually interactive way at a higher level of visual processing. The interaction (between, say, color and motion) would be recorded by a relative adaptation across a bank of neurons at the higher level. Thereafter the activation of this system by either of the original sets of neurons could re-create the impression of adaptation in the other set, thereby yielding the appropriate negative aftereffect.

This account still relies on the notion of adaptation, or habituation, of neurons. These hypothetical neurons, however, are at least removed from the feature-analyzing neurons that have been studied intensively and have not been observed to exhibit long-term adaptation effects. Neurons of this kind, which store patterns of interaction by means of long-term habituation, may play a rather general role in learning and memory.

appear to rotate in the direction in which the spiral was previously seen rotating and a colorless vertical grating employed to test for the McCollough effect would appear green if the vertical orientation had been paired with green. The striking feature of negative aftereffects, however, is that when two attributes are combined in a stimulus, one of them subsequently becomes associated with an opposite quality of the other (movement in the other direction, the complementary color and so on).

It is plausible that fatigue could become associated with aspects of the adapting stimulus, since it is known that the processes of fatigue start operating as soon as one looks at a stimulus. When one views something that is constantly moving, the perceived velocity decreases. When one looks at a colored surface, the color appears to become desaturated. (The reader can verify this relation by looking at one of the colored patches in the illustration on page 54. If half of the patch is obscured by a piece of gray paper that is removed after about 30 seconds, the part of the patch that was covered appears to be brighter than the part that was exposed.)

We have now examined two possible explanations of negative aftereffects: fatigue and conditioned fatigue. Possibly they both play a role. Masland's work on the spiral aftereffect showed that it has two components. One of us (Favreau) has conducted experiments that suggest a further dissociation of the short- and long-term components of this aftereffect. The simple aftereffect is observable immediately after one looks at a spiral, and it also decreases steadily in strength. The color-contingent spiral aftereffect is not seen immediately and does not reach full strength for several minutes. The finding suggests that during an exposure to spirals of alternating motion and colors, visual units sensitive to both directions of motion may be-

come fatigued and hence prevent the rapid appearance of a motion aftereffect. As the fatigue wears off, the effects of mechanisms underlying the color contingency may be revealed.

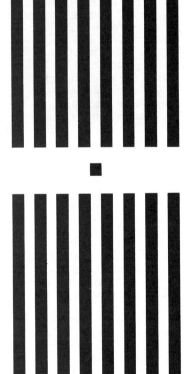

SPATIAL VARIATIONS can also cause aftereffects, apparently because certain neurons in the visual system are sensitive to spatial frequencies, that is, the spacing of more or less regular features of something one is looking at. One can obtain the aftereffect by first looking at the two sets of vertical bars at the left to determine whether they are the same. Then move your eyes back and forth along the horizontal bar between the two sets of vertical bars for about five minutes. When you shift your gaze to the horizontal bar between the vertical grids at the right, the spatial frequency of the grid at the top will appear to be higher than that of the grid at the bottom. If the illustration is turned upside down, the spatial relations will then reverse.

6

The Perception of Moving Targets

by Robert Sekuler and Eugene Levinson
January 1977

Highly specialized nerve circuits enable the human visual system to separate information about the direction in which an object is moving from the details of the object's pattern

The ability to respond promptly and appropriately to a moving object is often a matter of life or death. Hence it is not surprising that the mammalian visual system has evolved highly specialized neural mechanisms to handle the job. Physiological experiments in which microelectrodes are implanted in the visual cortex of an animal's brain have provided investigators with a wealth of information about how this complex nerve circuitry works in various species. In order to study the corresponding function in man, however, less invasive techniques are obviously required. Although the procedures developed for the latter purpose are necessarily indirect, they have yielded some striking information about the mechanisms employed by the human visual system to perceive moving objects.

The first requirement of any such psychophysical procedure is the provision of special stimuli. The moving things one sees in everyday life are not very helpful here, because their impact on the visual system is both too complicated and too weak to be measured reliably. Therefore even though the ultimate objective is of course to understand why moving objects appear the way they do in everyday life, one must start by working with moving targets that are both less complicated and more powerful than ordinary objects.

As far back as early in the 19th century students of human visual perception realized that prolonged exposure to a simple, strong stimulus could reveal properties of the motion-perception system that could not be observed with more variable stimuli. The British investigator R. Addams, for example, noted that prolonged fixation on motion in one direction often resulted in a peculiar aftereffect. Addams stared at a waterfall near Loch Ness for several seconds. When he then shifted his gaze to the rocks next to the waterfall, the rocks seemed to move upward. Earlier the Czech physiologist Jan Purkinje had experienced a similar illusion after watching a parade of horseback riders for about an hour.

In our laboratory at Northwestern University we obtain comparable effects by means of electronically generated stimuli. One kind of stimulus we find useful consists of a moving pattern of small, bright dots "painted" on the screen of a cathode-ray tube with the aid of a computer. The dots are usually distributed across the screen in a random fashion. Opposite sides of the screen are functionally connected: when a dot disappears off one side of the screen, it immediately reappears at the other. From the point of view of an observer it is as though he were looking at an infinitely large sheet of dots moving behind a stationary aperture. Because the dots are distributed randomly on the sheet, they enable us to study the visual impact of their motion without the complicating effects of perceived contours.

Another suitable kind of target, also created on a cathode-ray tube, is a pattern of alternating dark and light parallel bars. Patterns of this type, called gratings, can be made to drift at any speed in a direction perpendicular to the bars. With either gratings or dot patterns we are able to generate movement that is continuous, repetitive and of any desired duration. The individual, momentary effect of the motion can be allowed to accumulate, producing a total impact large enough to be measured reliably.

For any target, including a moving one, the response of the visual system depends on the contrast between the dark and light parts of the image. The fact that a television set has separate controls for contrast and brightness serves as a reminder that the two variables are not the same. At any level of average brightness one can independently adjust the contrast, making the picture more or less "washed out." In order to measure how effectively a certain television image stimulates the visual system, one possible approach is to adjust the contrast until an observer can barely see that the television screen is not perfectly uniform in its luminance. If the particular image on the screen happens to be one to which the observer

is very sensitive, it will remain visible even at a very low contrast.

It follows that the contrast threshold at which a target image disappears can be utilized as an index of an observer's sensitivity to that particular target. A low contrast threshold would mean a high sensitivity and vice versa. The same approach can be taken with an electronically generated grating or dot pattern: by reducing the contrast until the observer can barely see the pattern one can obtain a measure of the observer's contrast threshold for that pattern.

Ulker T. Keesey of the University of Wisconsin and Janos Kulikowski of the University of Manchester have shown that for many moving targets observers have not one but two distinct contrast thresholds. Suppose, for example, one is working with a low-frequency grating (that is, one with wide bars) moving across the screen of a cathode-ray tube. One starts with the contrast at zero and then gradually increases it until the observer can just detect that something is present. The observer does not actually see the grating; what he perceives is a procession of formless ripples. Although he can determine the direction in which the ripples are moving, the bars of the grating are themselves indistinct. If one now increases the contrast further, the bars too become visible. Evidently at a very low contrast a target's motion may be visible even though the characteristics of its pattern are not, whereas at a somewhat higher contrast both the pattern and its motion are discernible. The existence of separate thresholds for the perception of motion and the perception of pattern leads quite naturally to the suspicion that within the human nervous system there are two separate visual channels for analyzing these two aspects of a moving target.

Obviously there are limits to how much one can learn about the nervous system's response to motion from just watching a moving target. More analytic tools are needed. One such tool, frequently employed to study smell, hearing and taste as well as vision, is the psychophysical procedure known as selective adaptation. This technique makes it possible to "dissect" any sensory system painlessly. In selective adaptation one compares the detection of various stimuli before and after exposing the sensory system to a strong level of a particular stimulus, termed the adapting stimulus. Imagine, say, that exposure to some adapting stimulus makes it hard to detect one test stimulus but has little or no effect on the ability to detect another test stimulus. It would be reasonable to conclude that the mechanisms needed to

detect the first test stimulus overlap the mechanisms affected by the adapting stimulus but that the mechanisms needed to detect the second test stimulus do not. The adapting stimulus is usually thought of as fatiguing, or reducing the sensitivity of, selected mechanisms in the nervous system; reduced sensitivity makes it more difficult to detect the stimuli that are processed by the affected mechanism.

About a dozen years ago selective-adaptation experiments established that at

some stage of neural processing the human visual system makes use of mechanisms that are directionally selective. Leo Ganz, who is now at Stanford University, and one of us (Sekuler) had observers view vertical gratings that moved either to the left or to the right. The adapting stimuli were of high contrast; they were designed to selectively desensitize mechanisms that responded to only one direction of motion or the other, if indeed such mechanisms existed. After a short adapting period con-

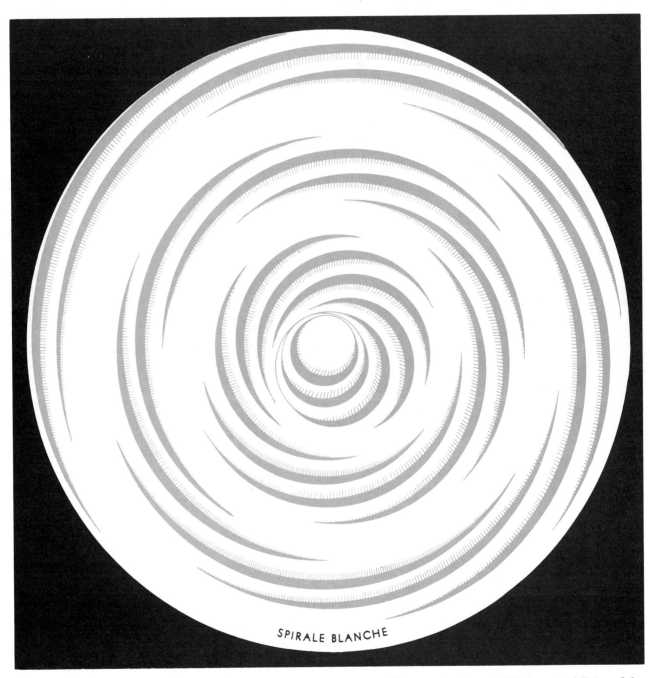

SPIRALE BLANCHE

"WHITE SPIRAL," one of a set of 12 rotating optical illusions called Rotoreliefs designed by the artist Marcel Duchamp in 1935, demonstrates an important property of the human visual system: the independence of the neural channels responsible for perceiving opposite directions of motion. When a copy of the design is rotated clockwise at a speed of about 33 revolutions per minute (on a phonograph turntable, say), a viewer should be able to see two superposed spirals: a dark one with many narrow turns, which appears to drift toward the center of rotation, and a white one with fewer, broader turns, which seems to move outward from the center. The two interwoven spiral patterns are actually fixed with respect to each other; nevertheless, when they are viewed in rotation (preferably with one eye), the two directions of motion separate clearly. This reproduction is from a set of Duchamp Rotoreliefs in the collection of Anne d'Harnoncourt.

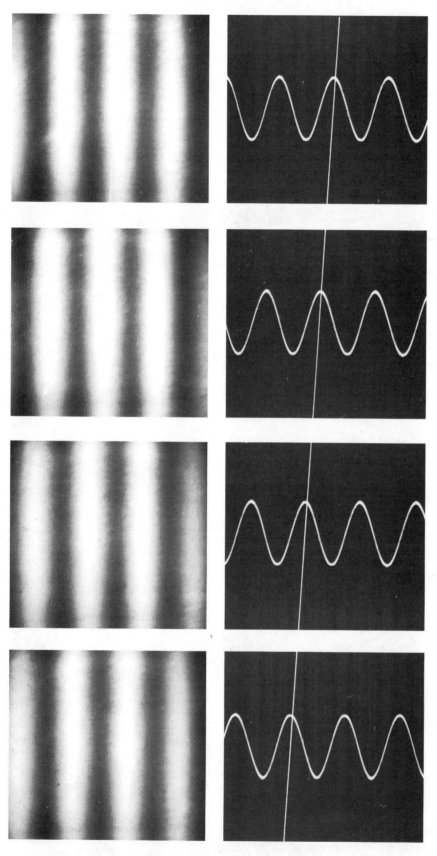

MOVING PATTERN of alternating dark and light parallel bars can be created on the screen of a cathode-ray tube in order to provide a suitable target for psychophysical experiments with human observers. In the sequence of photographs at the left, made in the authors' laboratory, a grating is shown drifting to the left across the screen at a constant rate. Sinusoidal curve associated with each photograph is a plot of light intensity across the screen at the moment of each exposure. Long slanted line connects a given peak on each curve at successive intervals.

trast thresholds were measured for a grating that moved either in the same direction as the adapting stimulus or in the opposite direction. There was a significant difference between the visibility of the two opposite directions of test movement: after adaptation it was much harder to see the grating that moved in the same direction as the adapting grating. This effect—called direction-specific adaptation—has been re-created many times since.

Naturally we wondered whether the mechanisms we were dealing with were related to single neural cells that show a strong preference for direction of motion. A directionally selective neuron discharges strongly when a properly oriented stimulus drifts in one direction through its visual field; it fires at a much reduced rate if the same stimulus moves through the field in the opposite direction. Direction-specific cells are abundant in the visual cortex of both the monkey and the cat. Because this kind of neuron is able to discriminate between directions of motion, it could provide the basis for the human ability to see moving targets. Although it is not certain that the human brain has exactly the same kinds of cells as a monkey's brain, it is known that in areas of vision not directly concerned with motion man's visual abilities are nearly identical with those of certain monkeys. Moreover, monkeys appear to experience motion aftereffects in much the same way that human beings do.

Several investigators have tried to determine whether or not the electrical activity of the human brain also shows directional selectivity. Electrodes can be fastened to an observer's scalp, and after proper amplification and signal processing the massed response from the brain tissue lying under the electrodes can be measured. The direction-specific adaptation experiment can then be done with the massed brain response. For example, one investigator measured the brain's response to a pattern moving first in one direction and then in the opposite direction. Adaptation produced a change in the brain's response to motion in the same direction as the adapting motion; the response to motion in the opposite direction was not affected.

Selective-adaptation experiments, in short, provide evidence that the human visual system contains some direction-selective mechanisms. The directional selectivity shown with adaptation techniques, however, does not tell one everything one would like to know about how the system responds to a moving stimulus. For example, the kind of selectivity observed in these experiments does not necessarily mean that there are separate detectors for opposite directions of motion. Direction-specific adaptation might reflect activity in directionally selective neurons whose outputs are subsequently pooled at a detection stage that is not direction-specific. Adaptation experiments confirm that the visual system analyzes direction of motion, but one would like to know how the information is treated after this preliminary analysis.

To test any system's ability to respond independently to either of two inputs, an engineer might examine how that system responds to the sum of the inputs. The basic idea is to compare the system's response to some stimulus alone with the system's response to the same stimulus when it is accompanied by an additional stimulus. If the presence of the additional stimulus neither helps nor hinders one's ability to detect the original target, the two stimuli would have to be detected by independent mechanisms.

We have exploited this approach in the following way. Starting with two separate cathode-ray tubes, on one we generate a grating that drifts to the right while on the other we produce a similar grating that drifts to the left. The images of the two tubes are combined optically (with a half-silvered mirror) and viewed by an observer, who adjusts the contrast of the combination grating to the threshold level.

Although we have made many measurements with the aid of this basic procedure, there is one special condition that is of particular interest: the case in which both gratings have the same bar width and contrast, drift at the same speed but move in opposite directions. In this case the combination stimulus shows neither direction of drift; it simply reverses repetitively in phase! At any one point on the observer's retina the combination grating changes from light to dark and back again, without any obvious drift in either direction. In fact, when an observer takes a quick look at such a high-contrast combination grating, he sees no movement; the grating simply appears to pulsate, with the dark bars getting light and vice versa.

Suppose now that an observer views one of the moving component gratings, adjusting its contrast until something is barely visible. He then repeats this procedure with the other moving component grating, also presented alone. The two thresholds will appear at about the same contrast value. Next the observer views the combination grating, always keeping the contrast of each moving component at its own threshold value. If gratings moving in opposite directions are detected independently, the combination grating would also be exactly at threshold. In order for the combination grating to be visible at all each of its oppositely moving components would require enough contrast to be visible in its own right. The actual appearance of the combination grating at the threshold level suggests that this line of reasoning is correct: when the combination is just

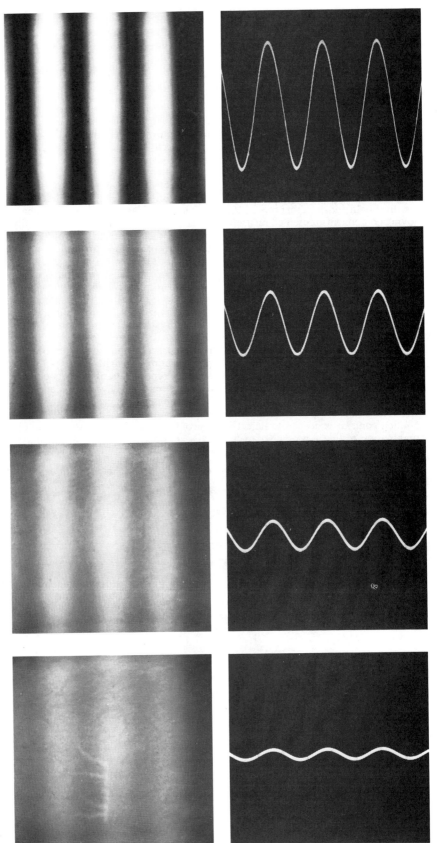

CONTRAST THRESHOLD, the level of contrast between the dark and light parts of a target image at which the image can barely be seen, serves as an index of an observer's sensitivity to that target. In the sequence of photographs at the left, for example, the contrast of four otherwise identical stationary gratings is progressively reduced from top to bottom. For moving targets human observers have been found to have two distinct contrast thresholds: one for perception of motion and the other for perception of pattern. Curves at right indicate light intensity.

at threshold, the observer sees first one and then the other component. The detection of the combination stimulus seems to depend on two independent visual mechanisms, each one responsible for detecting just one directional component, and these mechanisms fluctuate slightly in sensitivity over time.

The possibility that oppositely moving components in a combination grating are detected by independent direction-sensitive mechanisms leads to an interesting prediction: The contrast threshold for detecting a combination grating should be exactly twice the contrast threshold for detecting one of the moving components presented by itself. One expects this twofold difference because, as we have already explained, if either component of the combination grating is at the contrast threshold, then both components are at the contrast threshold, giving the combination grating as a whole a total contrast of two threshold units. Accordingly in our experiments we have compared the contrast threshold for a combination grating with the contrast threshold for either of its moving grating components presented alone, repeating the measurements at different bar widths and drift rates. The results are unequivocal: twice as much contrast is needed to detect a combination grating as is required to detect one of the moving grating components of the combination stimulus.

Since the combination grating made of oppositely moving components of equal contrast is so important in the study of vision, it has been given a special name: counterphase, or phase-alternating, grating. To examine other uses of the counterphase grating, we can start by relating our psychophysical results to some recent studies of single neurons in the cat's visual cortex. John G. Robson and Graham Cooper of the University of Cambridge have recorded the responses of single cells to unidirectional moving gratings and to counterphase gratings. A cell that responds equally well to either direction of grating drift discharges as strongly to a counterphase grating as it does to a moving grating of the same contrast. A cell that is directionally selective, however, responds about half as well to a counterphase grating as it does to an equal-contrast moving grating. The direction-selective cell, then, seems to respond only to the half-contrast component of the counterphase grating that drifts in the cell's preferred direction. Parallel psychophysical measurements have been made with cats: relying on a behavioral technique, John M. Camisa, Randolph Blake and one of us (Levinson) have found that the cat's contrast threshold for a counter-

phase grating is twice as high as it is for a unidirectional moving grating. These results are similar to our psychophysical observations with human subjects.

The twofold difference between the contrast thresholds for counterphase gratings and unidirectional moving gratings is not the only reason for believing the human visual system decomposes the counterphase grating into its separate moving components. Prior adaptation to a grating moving in one direction can radically alter the appearance of a counterphase grating. If, for example, one stares at a grating moving to the left—thereby desensitizing mechanisms sensitive to leftward motion—a subsequently seen counterphase grating initially appears to drift to the right. After several seconds the grating again assumes its normal pulsating appearance. Presumably the time during which the counterphase grating appears to drift to the right is the time during which the leftward-selective channel is less sensitive than the rightward-selective channel. As the effect of adaptation decays, the sensitivities of the channels regain parity and the pulsating appearance returns. It does seem somewhat peculiar that the visual system can extract the two moving components from a stimulus that hides movement as well as a counterphase grating does. Similar ex-

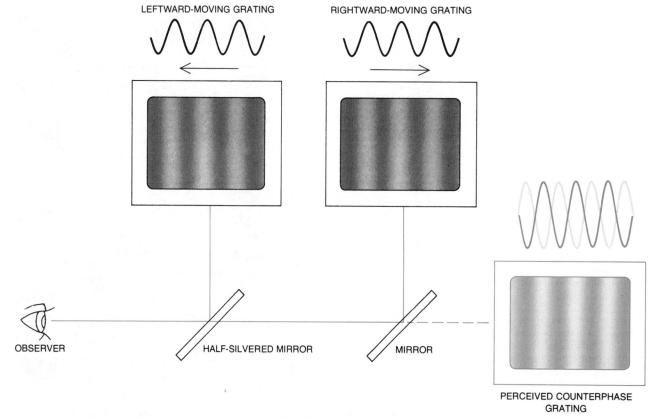

COUNTERPHASE GRATING, also known as a phase-alternating grating, is made by combining two oppositely moving gratings that have the same bar width and contrast. In the experimental setup shown here two separate cathode-ray tubes are used; on one the grating moves to the right while on the other the grating moves to the left. The images on the two tubes are combined optically with a half-silvered mirror and are viewed by an observer. The resulting visual stimulus (color) shows neither direction of drift; it simply reverses repetitively in phase. Nevertheless, the eye can readily decompose flickering image into its two oppositely moving component images.

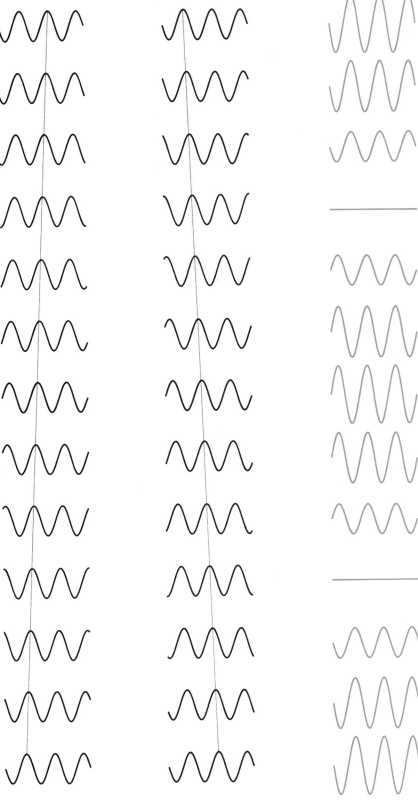

tractions are known, however, in other sensory domains. The decomposition into moving components is reminiscent of the ear's ability to separate a chord into its individual harmonic tones.

The ability of the visual system to use independent detectors to analyze a complex moving pattern into its components is no more surprising than the ability of the system to perform the reverse operation: the synthesis of such a pattern from its components. To demonstrate this synthesizing ability we presented a leftward-moving grating to one eye and a rightward-moving grating of equal contrast to the other eye, allowing the observer's brain to combine the two. The resulting synthetic percept was identical with a counterphase grating that could have been created by combining the two moving gratings with a half-silvered mirror. This synthesis reinforces the idea that the visual system can put complex patterns together as well as take them apart.

Most of the work we have discussed so far has focused on the role of human neural mechanisms in detecting motion, that is, in determining whether or not a moving target is visible. A more difficult and intriguing problem remains: the contribution of such mechanisms to the appearance of moving targets that are clearly visible. Our recent work at Northwestern shows that an observer's immediate perceptual history determines not only whether a moving target will be visible but also how the target will look if it does become visible. For example, we have found that adaptation to a sheet of random dots drifting uniformly in one direction can drastically change the apparent direction of subsequently viewed moving test dots. The shift in the perceived direction, which can be as much as 10 degrees of arc, is maximal when the adapting direction and the test direction are similar; the resulting shift is always away from the adapting direction. This direction shift is easily understood if one assumes that the neural code for perceived direction depends on a set of direction-specific mechanisms, each tuned to a somewhat different direction. The dots in the adapting pattern change the pattern of responsiveness among the mechanisms, thereby altering the apparent direction of the test stimulus.

It is now clear that with low-level stimulation at the contrast threshold the visual system decomposes complex stimuli and responds to each of the components without interference from the others. These separation processes do not tell the whole story, however. In everyday situations most stimuli are far above the contrast threshold and as a result the visual system's operation changes: interactions rather than independent responses are the rule, and the interactions tend to be inhibitory.

DECOMPOSITION OF A COUNTERPHASE GRATING into two oppositely moving gratings is represented graphically. The first column shows successive light-intensity curves for a sinusoidal grating drifting to the left at a constant rate. The second column shows the corresponding curves for a similar grating drifting to the right at the same rate. Each of the colored curves in the third column gives the algebraic sum of the other two curves in the same row; the curves in this column, representing the counterphase grating, go through one complete cycle of phase reversal in the 12 sampled time intervals. The peak-to-peak amplitude of the top curve in the third column is twice the amplitude of either of the other two curves in that row. This ratio is symbolic of the fact that the contrast threshold for detecting a counterphase grating is exactly twice contrast threshold for detecting either of two components presented by itself.

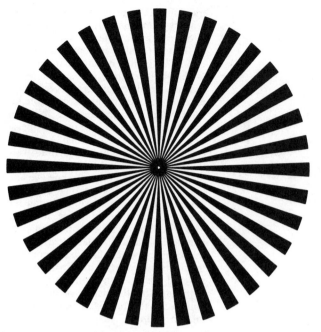

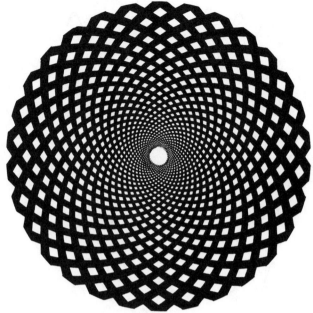

NEGATIVE AFTEREFFECT in the perception of motion can be demonstrated with these two designs. Place a copy of the radial "adapting" pattern at the left on a phonograph turntable. Stare at the center of the pattern as it spins at a speed of $33\frac{1}{3}$ r.p.m. Then look at the center of the stationary pattern at the right. The second pattern will briefly appear to be rotating in opposite direction. Experiments conducted with electronically generated moving stimuli reveal similar adaptation effects (*see bottom illustration on next page*).

To see how such inhibition works we turn to the horseshoe crab *Limulus polyphemus*. A great deal is known about the inhibitory activity in the faceted eye of *Limulus*. If one photoreceptor in that eye is strongly illuminated and a neighboring receptor is weakly illuminated, for example, the more strongly illuminated receptor reduces the neighbor's response. The inhibition is reciprocal: each photoreceptor can inhibit its neighbors and be inhibited by them. The net mutual inhibition depends on the relative strength of the illumination and the proximity of the photoreceptors to one another.

One important feature of such inhibition is that it does not operate all the time. For example, in the *Limulus* eye there are levels of illumination that are adequate to stimulate a photoreceptor but are inadequate to make that photoreceptor inhibit any of its neighbors. In order for inhibition to become apparent, stimulation must be increased. Thus at low levels of stimulation each receptor acts as an independent entity, whereas at higher levels of stimulation inhibitory interactions show up.

What role might inhibition play in human motion perception? Fred Attneave of the University of Oregon has pointed to the possible role of inhibition in various reversible or multistable figures. He cites the Necker cube, a visual illusion that seems to flip back and forth between orientations, as a good example of this phenomenon. There are reversible figures in motion perception too, and the counterphase grating is one of them. We mentioned above that a counterphase grating appears to pulsate or

flicker when it is briefly viewed. When a low-frequency counterphase grating is observed for a longer time, however, its appearance changes in a way that is reminiscent of the alterations of more common reversible figures. The counterphase grating sometimes seems to drift in one direction and then in the other. The grating produces a multistable percept, and multistability, as Attneave has shown, is a symptom of inhibition [see "Multistability in Perception," by Fred Attneave; SCIENTIFIC AMERICAN, December, 1971].

We have also made more objective measurements of reciprocal inhibition between channels tuned to opposite directions of motion. In one experiment we measured the contrast threshold for a rightward-moving grating after adaptation to two different kinds of stimulus. One was simply a rightward-moving grating; the other was a combination of that same rightward-moving grating with a leftward-moving one. We knew that the rightward-adapting grating by itself would decrease the visibility of a test grating moving in the same direction. We wanted to determine whether an added leftward component could reduce the effectiveness of the rightward-adapting stimulus. If adding increasing amounts of the leftward component produces more inhibition, the adapting power of the rightward component should be reduced. As it turns out, that is exactly what happens.

Work on the physiology of motion sensitivity in lower animals complements our observations on inhibition in human motion-perception mecha-

nisms. In general inhibition serves the function of "neural sharpening"; in other words, it accentuates the differences between a mechanism's responses to different stimuli. The responses of directionally selective neurons in the visual cortex of the cat to their nonpreferred directions of movement are often lower than the maintained, unstimulated activity of those cells. A number of investigators have recently shown that this reduction in response can sometimes be eliminated after administration of the drug bicuculline, an antagonist for the putative inhibitory neurotransmitter gamma-aminobutyric acid. In this case inhibition increases the difference between a neuron's responses to motion in its preferred and its nonpreferred directions and thereby improves the directional selectivity.

Inhibition between direction-specific units is apparently weak at birth and its development requires some visual experience. John D. Pettigrew, now at the California Institute of Technology, has found a lack of inhibition in the visual response to movement in the nonpreferred direction in the cortex of a newborn cat or a visually deprived adult cat. Consistent with this observation are experiments reported by Max Cynader at Dalhousie University. Cynader and his colleagues raised cats in a visual environment in which the cats were exposed to only one direction of motion. The vast majority of direction-selective cortical neurons of these "unidirectional" cats preferred movement in the direction to which the cats had been exposed during rearing. This bias in direction preference contrasts sharply with the

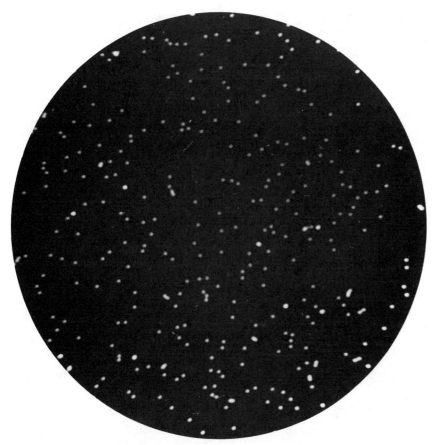

SPECIAL STIMULUS employed by the authors in their laboratory to study the perception of motion under controlled conditions consists of a moving pattern of small, bright dots electronically generated on the screen of a cathode-ray tube with a computer. To an observer the stimulus looks like an infinitely large sheet of random dots moving behind a stationary aperture.

comparatively uniform distribution of direction preference in normally reared cats. Although it is not yet known what perceptual deficits might accompany this abnormal distribution of direction preference, it is clear that the physiological characteristics of motion-perception mechanisms depend critically on the kind of visual world the young cat experiences. One can speculate that

man's comparatively uniform sensitivity to different directions of movement might result from frequent exposure to all directions during infancy.

We mentioned above that there might be separate visual channels for analyzing the movement characteristics and the pattern characteristics of a stimulus. We have recently established that of these separate channels only those con-

cerned with motion show directional selectivity. When we measured the contrast thresholds for both motion perception and pattern perception after adaptation to movement in one direction, we found that the motion thresholds were raised more when the test stimulus and the adapting stimulus moved in the same direction than when they moved in opposite directions. Pattern thresholds, however, were equal for all test directions. In other words, although the adapting stimulus was exerting a strong directionally selective effect on the motion-perception system, it was having no directional effect on the pattern-perception system.

These observations suggest that the neural mechanism for detecting motion is independent of the mechanism for detecting pattern. Many other experiments support this view. We have already noted that the motion and pattern aspects of a moving target may have different contrast thresholds. Allan Pantle of the University of Miami has differentiated the two mechanisms in another way, by comparing their respective responses to variations in contrast. He relied on various procedures to determine how human direction-sensitive mechanisms respond to variation in the contrast of a moving target. All the procedures agreed: the two mechanisms have a very limited range of response to stimulus contrast. Their response increases linearly with the logarithm of stimulus contrast in the low-contrast region, but it is essentially independent of stimulus contrast once the contrast exceeds the threshold level by more than a factor of five or six. The response of the pattern-sensitive mechanisms does not appear to saturate at low contrast.

Additional evidence for the separation of the two systems comes from the examination of cases of brain pathology. Whitman A. Richards of the Massachusetts Institute of Technology has begun to accumulate evidence that some people who have normal pattern vision have difficulty seeing certain kinds of movement. Whether or not the difficulties are genetically determined remains to be seen, but the specificity of the loss is consistent with the idea of specialized machinery for the perception of motion. Moreover, certain kinds of neural damage (caused by gunshot wounds to the head, for instance) can result in a blind region in the visual field, called a scotoma. Observations of people with such neurological damage show that in areas of the visual field where stationary contours cannot be seen some residual sensitivity to moving stimulation is preserved.

A scotoma is often ignored by the person who has it; the visual system apparently extrapolates from the areas surrounding the functionally deficient region and fills it in with whatever the intact adjacent areas see. A dramatic new

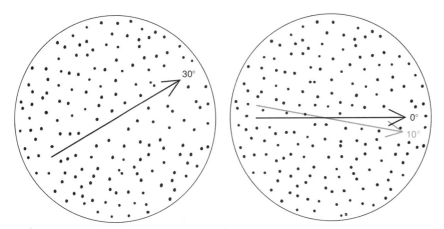

ADAPTATION TO A SHEET OF RANDOM DOTS drifting uniformly in one direction (*pattern at left*) can drastically change the apparent direction of a subsequently viewed sheet of moving test dots (*pattern at right*). The shift in the perceived direction (*colored arrow*) can be as large as 10 degrees of arc. The resulting shift is invariably away from adapting direction.

form of extrapolation in normal observers that depends on a moving stimulus was recently discovered in our laboratory by Paul Tynan and one of us (Sekuler). To demonstrate this completion effect a grating with a low spatial frequency is made to drift slowly across a cathode-ray tube. A section of opaque black construction paper, roughly half the height of the screen, is taped across the middle of the screen from one side to the other. Since the paper is opaque, none of the grating can actually be seen in the region covered by the paper. Nevertheless, a normal observer who stares at the center of the black paper will not see grating sections at top and bottom with a middle part missing; instead he will see a grating covering the entire field! The middle, illusory part is a good deal dimmer in overall luminance than the top and bottom parts, but it will be seen quite vividly. These moving "phantoms" appear to travel at the same speed and in the same direction as the pattern that induces them. They are different in this respect from other well-known illusions of motion. Moreover, very small strips of moving pattern separated by large distances are able to produce vivid phantom gratings extending across the entire blank space between them. If the grating stops drifting, the phantom section disappears. The illusion, which can also be created with a rotating radial grating, requires movement of the real grating sections [see illustration on this page].

Floyd Ratliff of Rockefeller University has suggested that the visual system might economize on the amount of data it transmits by extrapolating information from certain select points in the visual field [see "Contour and Contrast," by Floyd Ratliff; SCIENTIFIC AMERICAN, June, 1972]. A highly repetitive pattern is therefore treated as though it covered the entire field, even when the pattern actually has gaps. If the information going to the brain were compressed and abbreviated for economy of transmission, the brain would have to fabricate much of our visual experience, working from scant clues. Redundancies in the visual world usually allow this fabrication to pass unnoticed, but illusions can result when certain unusual stimuli are compressed and then reconstructed. The moving phantoms may clarify the nature of the extrapolation process.

Although the visual system normally discards some of the information it receives, the lack of certain forms of information will seriously degrade its performance. The mathematical theory of the "ideal detector" shows that if an observer does not know what target to expect, and where and when to expect it, he cannot detect the target as easily as he could if he had that knowledge. The ideal detector represents the best detection performance any sensory system can achieve; failure to reach that level can

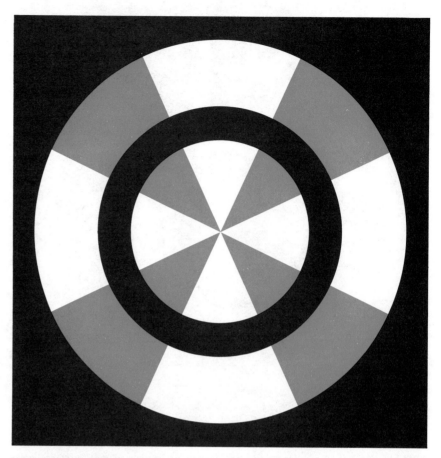

PHANTOM-CONTOUR EFFECT, a form of visual extrapolation in normal observers that depends on a moving stimulus, was discovered recently at Northwestern by one of the authors (Sekuler) and his colleague Paul Tynan. When one stares at the center of this radial pattern as it rotates on a phonograph turntable at 33$\frac{1}{3}$ r.p.m., one will see dim but distinct contours filling in the dark, blank region that interrupts the pattern. The phantom contours, which move in phase with their real neighbors, are enhanced by viewing the spinning disk in dim light.

provide clues about a sensory system's operation. With this possibility in mind Karlene Ball and one of us (Sekuler) have compared the detectability of dim, moving dots under two conditions: when the direction of movement was kept constant and when the direction of movement varied unpredictably from trial to trial. The observer's uncertainty about the direction of movement produced a dramatic loss in detectability. Analogous results have been obtained with uncertainty about the velocity of a target's motion. By examining the effect of various kinds and amounts of uncertainty we have improved our estimates of the direction-tuning and velocity-tuning functions of motion-sensitive mechanisms. Moreover, work with stimulus uncertainty provides a bridge between laboratory data and the motion perception of everyday life, in which stimulus uncertainty is pervasive and serious enough to play a major limiting role.

The effects we have observed with moving visual stimuli resemble analogous effects in other senses. Accordingly, although the perception of motion has interesting and unique properties of its own, the study of this particular ability is also valuable for what it reveals about vision and the other senses more generally. Other visual abilities, for example, seem to make use of coordinated mechanisms, each designed to do a particular job. In the human eye exquisite sensitivity to just a few photons of light coexists with excellent spatial resolving power. This coexistence is made possible in part by the operation of two classes of retinal photoreceptors: the rods and the cones. Similar divisions of labor are known in touch, hearing and taste.

It makes a good deal of sense for the human visual system to separate information about pattern and motion, and about different directions of motion as well. Often during the evolution of our species it must have been much more important to respond to the direction in which some poorly defined form moved than to appreciate the details of that form. Any pedestrian who has dodged traffic in a large city appreciates this fact and should be thankful that the mechanisms for motion perception and pattern perception can coexist in a way that enables each to do what it alone does best.

7

Hidden Visual Processes

by Jeremy M. Wolfe
February 1983

Vision is usually regarded as being a single sense.
Experiments show, however, that the visual system
includes subsystems whose operation is normally
hidden from the awareness of the perceiver

From the standpoint of a person contemplating his abilities to perceive the world, vision seems to be a single sense. The images impinging on the two retinas give rise to a single awareness of the objects in the world: their sizes, shapes, colors, textures and positions. This view, however, is mistaken. The visual system (the brain mechanism that processes data from the eyes) is actually a set of specialized subsystems each of which acts more or less independently on some subset of visual data. Furthermore, some of the visual subsystems have an output that cannot be seen. They contribute to brain function and even to our awareness of the world, but no amount of introspection can make us aware of the subsystems themselves. They perform hidden visual processes.

How is a hidden process revealed? One way is to examine the abilities of people who have suffered brain injury. Consider the pupil of the eye, which constricts in response to an increase in the intensity of light falling on the retina. If someone suffers an injury that destroys the visual cortex (the part of the cerebral cortex first in line to get data from the eyes), he is rendered perceptually blind. That is, his awareness of a loss of vision is the same as that of someone who has lost the use of the eyes themselves. Nevertheless, the pupils continue to constrict in response to light. Even more strikingly, Ernest C. Poppel, Richard Held and Douglas Frost of the Massachusetts Institute of Technology have found that when people who are perceptually blind because of an injury to the cerebral cortex are asked to direct their eyes toward a spot of light, they do surprisingly well. The subjects report that they cannot see the spot, and so they think they are guessing, but they look in roughly the right direction more often than chance would allow.

Brain-injured people thus show evidence of multiple visual processes: some that are damaged, and hidden ones that remain functional. What such studies cannot confirm is that similar hidden processes operate in people whose visual system is intact. For that, special experimental strategies are required. Here I shall describe three sets of experiments each of which reveals a visual process that in normal people is hidden from introspection. In this regard all of us are like the brain-injured patient who can look at a spot of light although he cannot perceive it. We too are unaware of the abilities of certain parts of the visual system even though our behavior is often based on their output.

One of the functions of the visual system is to control the muscles that focus the eye on objects at various distances by changing the shape of the lens. The closer the object is, the more nearly spherical the lens must be. The process is called visual accommodation. One's impression is that one can accommodate for anything one can see. It is natural to assume, therefore, that accommodation and visual perception have access to the same set of stimuli.

Do they? By means of a number of experimental methods the accommodative status of the eye can be measured while the subject looks at a stimulus placed a certain distance from him. In one such method the subject views the stimulus through polarizing filters, and a flash of light from behind a slit briefly superposes on the stimulus a bright horizontal bar. The filters have no effect on the stimulus, but they ensure that light from the left half of the bar will enter only the top of the lens of the subject's eye and light from the right half will enter only the bottom.

Suppose a subject who is looking at the stimulus is accommodating for a distance greater or less than the distance to the slit. If the bar is flashed at that instant, the two halves of it will be misaligned on the retina and the subject will see them as being offset. Hence the experimenter need only have the subject look at the stimulus while the bar repeatedly appears and ask the subject whether or not its halves are aligned. The slit is moved to various distances until the subject reports that they are aligned. The distance from the slit to the eye is then the distance for which the subject is accommodating.

The lens of the eye hardens with age, and so it is best to study accommodation in subjects no older than their 30's. In the laboratory such subjects can be shown stimuli that change only in distance, not in brightness and size. This eliminates all perceptual clues to the distance of the stimulus except the fact that a certain accommodative state brings the stimulus to a focus. Under these circumstances the typical subject's accommodation is about 90 percent of perfect. (If it were perfect, a stimulus at a distance of 25 centimeters would cause the eye to accommodate for a distance of 25 centimeters and so on.)

How does the eye respond when the stimulus has no features for the eye to focus on? One such stimulus would be a blank screen surrounding the subject; the experience is like being inside a giant ping-pong ball. Another stimulus would be a smaller blank screen viewed through a lens that makes the screen appear too close (in optical, or apparent, distance) for the eye to focus on its edges. Another would be a featureless sky; still another would be complete darkness. Herschel W. Leibowitz and D. Alfred Owens of Pennsylvania State University have found that in any of these circumstances the lens of the eye assumes a rather stable resting curvature for a particular focal distance called the dark focus. Each individual has a characteristic dark focus that is usually about one meter, or about an arm's length from the eye.

The same thing happens when the stimulus is a grating of black and white lines so fine that they give the impression of a gray field. Here again the experimenter's lens can place the stimulus at a variety of optical distances. When the stimulus is at an optical distance of 25 centimeters, the lens of the subject's eye assumes its resting state. When the stimulus is moved to an optical distance of one meter, the subject's accommodative state shows no change. The conclu-

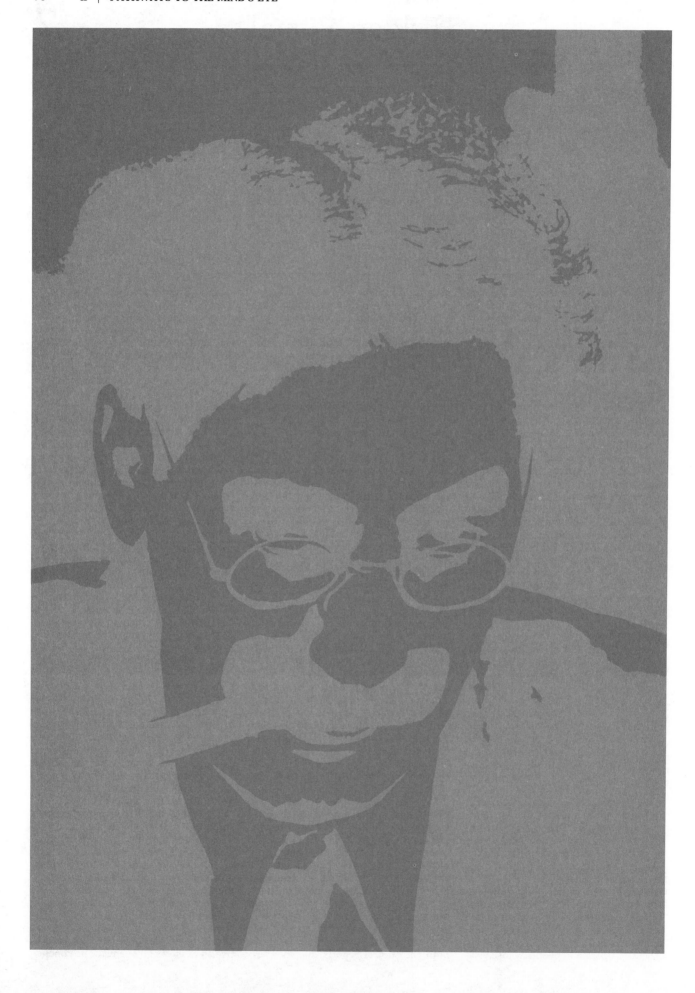

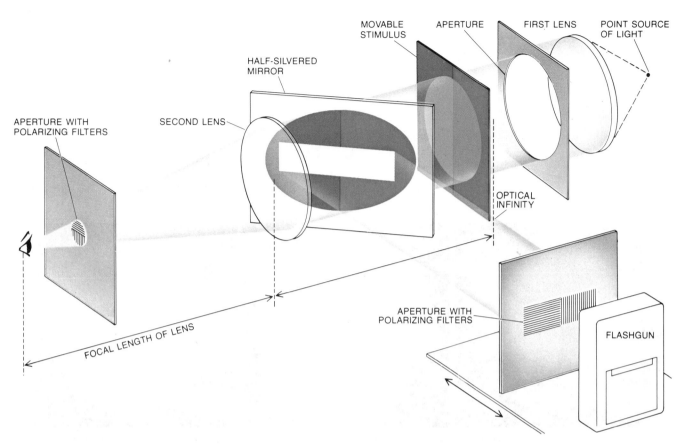

EXPERIMENTAL APPARATUS tests the ability of the eye to accommodate for an edge in an isoluminant stimulus. The lens toward the upper right in the illustration collimates a beam of light. The beam passes through an aperture, then through the stimulus, which has a vertical edge defined only by the colors red and green. A second lens directs light into the subject's eye. A further arrangement consisting of a flashgun, a movable slit and a half-silvered mirror briefly superposes on the isoluminant stimulus a horizontal bar of light.

sion is that accommodation can shape the lens of the eye to keep an object in focus only if the system responsible for accommodation is presented with something it can "see."

Armed with the knowledge that the accommodation system is blind to certain aspects of the visual world, Owens and I asked whether the system can "see" color. We measured accommodation while our subjects looked at a simple stimulus: a circular field divided vertically in half so that it included a single vertical edge. An optical system known as Maxwellian-view optics ensured that the perimeter of the circle was beyond optical infinity. That is, the rays of light from each point on the perimeter of the circle were made to enter the eye in such a way that they could never be brought into focus whatever

shape the lens of the eye assumed. As a result the vertical edge between the two halves of the field was really the only edge in the stimulus for which the eye could accommodate. The optical system was also designed to ensure that the image of the stimulus would keep the same size on the retina when we changed its optical distance.

The edge itself could be created by a difference in either color or brightness between the two half fields. In the real world most contours arise from a difference in both. We chose to make one half field red, the other green. Then we varied the brightness of one half field or the other. In this way we created stimuli ranging from an edge between red and black to an edge between black and green. At each extreme the contrast in brightness across the edge between the color and the black was 100 percent. In

the precisely intermediate case, however, the red and the green were equally bright. They formed an isoluminant stimulus whose single edge was defined only by color. The contrast in brightness was zero.

When we tested people's ability to accommodate for each of these stimuli, we found the ability declined as the contrast in brightness declined. Thus our subjects could readily tell that the isoluminant stimulus was an edge between red and green, but it was impossible for them to bring the edge into focus. In one experiment we had subjects look at a black *E* on a white background. The subjects accommodated quite well for optical distances from infinity down to 22 centimeters. Then we had them look at edges between red and black or between black and green. Their accommodation was about 80 percent as good as the best they had done for the *E*. Finally we showed them the red-green edge that has no contrast in brightness. Their accommodation was only 19 percent as good. When we repeated the experiment with pairs of colors such as red and orange or blue and green, the subjects' performance was equally poor or worse.

Like any other optical system, the eye has a chromatic aberration, which brings different colors to a focus at slightly different focal lengths. The ab-

ISOLUMINANT STIMULUS is an image whose edges are defined only by a change in color, not by a change in brightness. The stimulus here is imperfect: the blue parts and the green parts of the image are only as nearly equal in brightness as they can be on the printed page. Moreover, the change in brightness beyond the edge of the page is apparent, and so is the fact that the reader is holding the magazine at reading distance. When such cues are removed under laboratory conditions, subjects faced with an isoluminant stimulus prove unable to bring its edges into focus. This deficiency contributes to making a familiar face hard to recognize. The experiment indicates that the brain process underlying visual accommodation (the focusing of the eyes) cannot "see" color; it is a hidden process distinct from the processes that lead to perception. The image shows Groucho Marx as he appeared in the motion picture *Horse Feathers*.

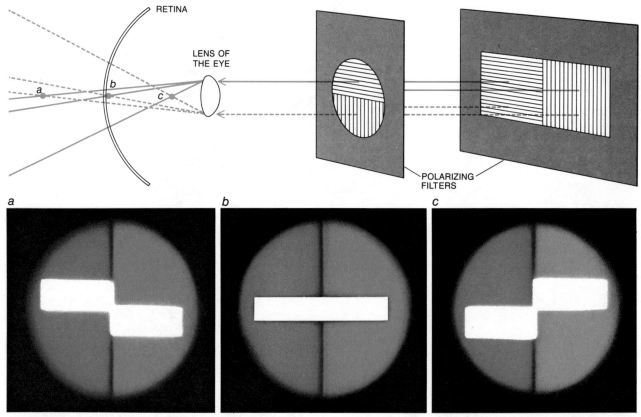

ACCOMMODATION IS MEASURED by having people describe the flashing horizontal bar. A series of polarizing filters ensures that light from the left side of the bar enters only the top of the lens of the subject's eye; light from the right side enters only the bottom. The two sides of the bar will line up on the retina (*b*) only if the subject happens to be accommodating for the distance to the movable slit.

erration therefore tends to shift the retinal image of one color half field with respect to the image of the other. This can give rise to a bright or dark contour depending on whether the images separate or overlap. As a result it is surprisingly difficult to create a stimulus that has absolutely no clues to the presence of an edge except the difference in color itself. We suspect our subjects' performance would have been even worse than it was if chromatic aberration could have been eliminated. Still, the conclusion seems clear: accommodation is colorblind, or at least it "sees" color very badly. It is a visual subsystem remarkably independent of visual perception. Here, then, is a finding that no amount of introspection could have suggested about vision.

A second strategy for exploring the division of the visual system into subsystems is to consider the ways a particular visual function is performed by different parts of the system. One such function is binocular vision. A normal person has two eyes, and the brain makes every effort to integrate the data from them. It is becoming clear, however, that the brain does more than simply combine the inputs from the eyes in one grand binocular process that leads to visual perception. Instead several special-purpose mechanisms combine the inputs in their own way to meet their own particular needs. Just as no amount of introspection will reveal that accommodation is colorblind, so no amount of introspection will reveal these multiple binocular processes. Nevertheless, the processes do exist and can be revealed by experimentation.

Consider a visual illusion that everyone has experienced in one form or another. You are sitting in a train, waiting for it to pull out of the station. Looking out the window, you see another train motionless on the adjacent track. The other train's image starts to slide backward, and you distinctly feel that your train is moving forward. Then you see it is the other train that has moved; your train is still in the station. The motion of the other train somehow deluded you into believing you were moving. You have experienced an illusion of motion created solely by visual stimulation. The illusion is known as vection.

Several investigators have sought to examine the brain mechanism responsible for vection. Held and I became interested in a rather different question. We wanted to know what the vection process can "see." In particular we wanted to know if the process can make use of peo-ple's ability to look at the world through two eyes. One might think the answer could be found quite easily by comparing the vection experienced when both eyes are open with the vection experienced when only one eye is open. Normally, however, the sensation of vection is already at its maximum when only one eye is open; the illusion of self-motion cannot be more pronounced. One needs, therefore, to create a stimulus whose binocular effect could conceivably be greater than its monocular effect. Such a stimulus must have a purely binocular component: there must be something about the stimulus that is invisible to each eye by itself.

A component that meets this requirement is called a cyclopean stimulus, after the Cyclops, the Homeric one-eyed creature encountered by Odysseus. The name is apt because a cyclopean stimulus is evident only if the brain combines the input from the eyes. In effect the brain must act as a single, cyclopean eye. One example of a cyclopean stimulus is the small difference in position between the image of an object in the world on each of the retinas. The difference can easily be seen. Stretch out one of your arms and look at the tip of a finger first with one eye closed and then with the other eye closed. You will notice that the two views are slightly different. The brain exploits such differences in the processes that lead to the perception of three-dimensional depth. Clearly the brain must draw on data from both eyes for the stimulus to exist.

Our cyclopean stimulus for vection capitalized on the well-known fact that objects seen in a motion picture seem to move smoothly even though they are presented in a succession of still photographs. Our subjects sat inside a cylinder three feet in diameter and five feet high. The inside surface of the cylinder was white and was covered with a random pattern of black dots an inch in diameter. The cylinder rotated about the subject at the rate of 30 degrees of angle per second. When the inner surface of the cylinder was illuminated by ordinary lighting, the subject reported a sensation of rotation in the opposite direction. For our experiments we illuminated the surface with the periodic flashes of a stroboscopic lamp. Each flash produced the equivalent of a frame from a movie of black dots. The subject reported the same sensation of vection.

To create a cyclopean stimulus two strobe lamps were needed. One was covered with a red filter, the other with a green filter. The subjects wore goggles that placed a red filter in front of one eye and a green filter in front of the other. No red light could pass through the green filter; no green light could pass through the red. Hence the light from one strobe lamp was seen by one eye and the light from the other strobe lamp was seen by the other eye.

Suppose each strobe lamp is flashing at 10 hertz, or 10 times per second. If the two lamps are flashing in phase (that is, in synchrony), the subject should notice no important difference in looking with two eyes rather than one. In either case he will see in effect a 10-frame-per-second movie of moving dots. Suppose, however, the strobe lamps are exactly out of phase, so that they flash in alternation. Now there is a difference. A subject who has only one eye open will see again a 10-frame-per-second movie. With both eyes open he will see an additional movie. It will appear at a rate of 20 frames per second, and it will consist of frames presented in alternation first to one eye, then to the other, then to the first eye again.

The 20-hertz interocular movie is thus a cyclopean stimulus: it cannot be seen by either eye alone. It does give rise to the appearance of motion. The question is whether the vection system can "see" it. If it can, the experiment where the strobe lamps are out of phase could produce a greater sensation of vection than the experiment where the lamps are in phase. If it cannot, the two experiments should have the same result.

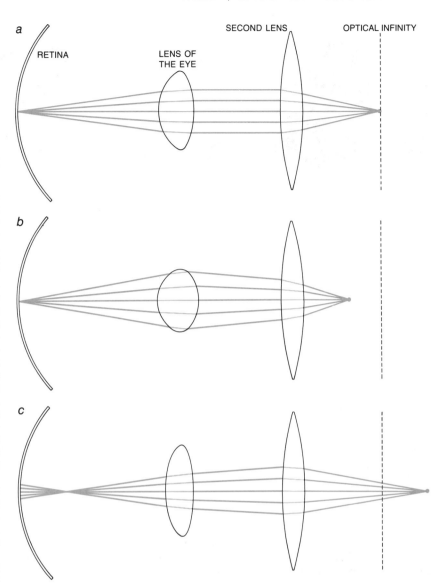

OPTICAL DISTANCE of a stimulus is the apparent distance given the stimulus by the second lens in the experimental apparatus. If the stimulus is positioned at the focal length of the lens (*a*), it will be at optical infinity, that is, the light rays from each part of the stimulus will approach the eye in parallel, as if they came from a source infinitely far away. The lens of the eye will assume a curvature that brings the rays to a point on the retina. If the stimulus is closer than optical infinity (*b*), the rays will diverge as they approach the eye. The lens of the eye will then assume a more nearly spherical shape to bring the rays to a focus. If the stimulus is farther away than optical infinity (*c*), the rays will converge as they approach the eye. The lens of the eye will be unable to reduce its curvature to the required extent; thus the rays will come to a point in front of the retina. A stimulus beyond optical infinity cannot be brought into focus.

With our apparatus in place we prepared subjects for the experiments. In particular we taught them a method known in experimental psychology as magnitude estimation. We asked them to give a rating of 10 to a compelling sensation of self-motion and one of zero to no sensation of motion. Ratings between 0 and 10 were to be given to sensations between these two extremes. Unlikely as it may seem, some 25 years of research in experimental psychology, notably the work of S. Smith Stevens of Harvard University, has shown that people are quite good at assigning numbers to their sensations. They can do it

repeatedly, systematically and reliably.

One thing did concern us: there could be no difference between the results of the two experiments if the sensation of vection yielded the maximum rating of 10 when the lamps were in phase. If the frames of a movie are shown at a progressively lower rate, the illusion of motion becomes progressively less compelling. In the same way the flicker rate turns out to be important to the sensation of self-motion. We found that any rate higher than about 2.5 hertz produced some degree of vection, but only rates higher than about 15 hertz consistently earned ratings of 10 from our sub-

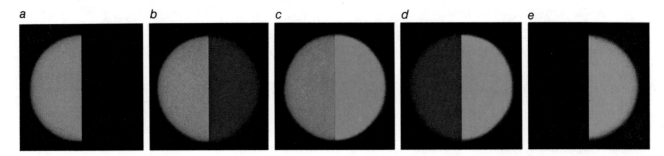

a   *b*   *c*   *d*   *e*

STIMULI FOR THE EXPERIMENT on the ability to accommodate vary from an edge between red and black (*a*) to an edge between black and green (*e*). The precisely intermediate stimulus (*c*) is isoluminant. The circular perimeter of each stimulus is defined by an aperture placed well beyond optical infinity in the experimental apparatus; hence the subject's eye cannot bring the perimeter into focus.

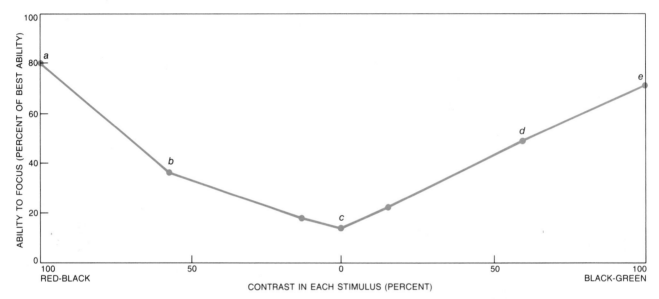

ABILITY TO FOCUS on the stimuli turns out to depend on their contrast in brightness. Here the average performance of four subjects is charted as a percentage of the ability they had when they looked at black letters on an eye-examination chart. The subjects' performance grows poorer with decreasing contrast. It is worst (19 percent of the best performance) when the stimulus is isoluminant.

jects. Therefore flicker rates between 2.5 hertz and 15 hertz would suit our purpose. The cyclopean stimulus created (at twice the flicker rate) by flashing the lamps out of phase would be capable in principle of producing a more compelling sensation of vection than the stimulus produced by leaving the lamps in phase.

Our findings were straightforward. For any flicker rate between 2.5 hertz and 15 hertz the two strobes out of phase always elicited the greater magnitude estimates. Evidently the vection system can "see" the purely binocular stimulus. Does this result establish that the brain has multiple binocular processes? Not in itself. As I have noted, the slight difference in position between the images of an object on each retina is a cyclopean clue to three-dimensional depth. It is conceivable that the binocular mechanism serving this aspect of visual perception also serves the binocular contribution to vection.

Some people, however, cannot perceive depth on the basis of cyclopean stimuli. For example, they cannot get the illusion of depth when they look at an image through a stereoscope or when they go to a "3-D" movie. They are stereoblind. Some of them are born that way, just as some people are born colorblind. Others lose the ability because of defects that develop in infancy in the ability to align the eyes. Stereoblindness is somewhat rarer than colorblindness; it seems to affect only a few percent of the U.S. population. A person who is stereoblind can still perceive depth on the basis of visual cues such as the apparent size of familiar objects or the fact that some objects in the visual field block others that are farther away. These monocular cues to three-dimensional depth are quite good; many people who are stereoblind do not know they are until a test reveals it.

Held and I asked four people who had been established as stereoblind to be subjects in our vection experiments. Their magnitude estimations were much like those of our normal subjects. They too got an increased sensation of self-motion from the purely binocular stimulus. Here, then, are people with a defective binocular mechanism who nonetheless prove to be perfectly normal in experiments requiring that their brain employ a binocular mechanism. Thus the defective mechanism cannot be the only binocular mechanism in the brain. There must be at least two binocular mechanisms, one mediating stereoscopic depth perception, the other involved in the production of vection. The experiments again show that visual data feed more than one processing system.

The two hidden visual processes I have now described (the colorblind visual process that controls accommodation and the binocular visual process that contributes to vection) appear to play no direct role in visual perception.

Other hidden visual processes do take part in perception.

For an example I shall return to the binocular visual processes. Our experiments with vection revealed two binocular processes. The experiments I shall now describe show more. Indeed, there emerges a remarkable assortment of processes. Between our two eyes and our single perception of the visual world lie processes that can "see" out of one eye, processes that can "see" out of either eye and, most surprising, a purely binocular process: a process that can "see" only out of both eyes. In fact, it can "see" only when both eyes are looking at the same stimulus. If your visual system had only the purely binocular process, you would be unable to see if one eye was closed. You would be un-able to see when you tried, for example, to peek out from behind a tree and one eye surveyed only tree bark while the other surveyed a house.

The ability to perceive a purely binocular stimulus such as the cyclopean stimulus that served our study of vection does not ensure that the brain has a purely binocular visual process. The cyclopean stimulus could have been "seen" by a visual process that accepts input from both eyes and also from either eye alone. How, then, is it known that a purely binocular process is there? Again one resorts to an indirect method, in this case based on a temporary distortion of vision called the tilt aftereffect.

Look at the pattern of stripes at the right in the illustration above. The top half of the pattern should appear to be aligned with the bottom half. Now look at the chevron pattern at the left in the illustration. Let your eyes scan back and forth for one or two minutes along the horizontal black bar that crosses the center of the chevron, then quickly shift your gaze to the pattern at the right. You should find that the two halves no longer seem aligned. They should appear to be bent in the direction opposite to the direction of the bend in the chevron.

This is the tilt aftereffect. It can be measured by making the two halves of the pattern at the right adjustable and asking people to make the two halves look aligned. Before people view the chevron they make settings quite close to colinearity. After viewing the chevron their settings are systematically displaced by about two degrees.

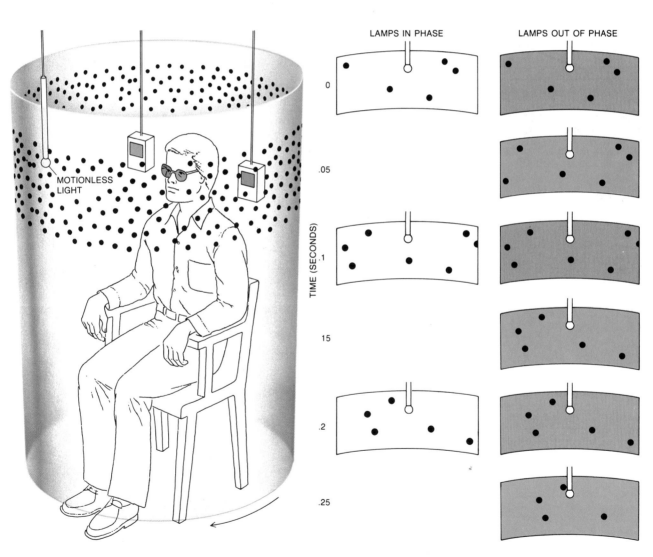

LAMPS IN PHASE   LAMPS OUT OF PHASE

TIME (SECONDS)

0
.05
.1
15
.2
.25

MOTIONLESS LIGHT

EXPERIMENT WITH VECTION (the sensation of bodily motion arising from the motion of the visual world) requires that subjects be seated inside a rotating cylinder whose inner surface is white and is covered with a random pattern of black dots. Two stroboscopic lamps illuminate the surface in flashes of red and green light; a pair of goggles allows the light of each color to enter one eye only. If the lamps flash in phase (that is, synchronously) at a rate of 10 flashes per second, a subject with one eye open sees what a subject with both eyes open sees: in effect a 10-frame-per-second motion picture of moving dots. If the lamps flash out of phase, a subject with one eye open sees the identical movie, but a subject with both eyes open sees an additional movie. It appears at a rate of 20 frames per second, and it is interocular: its successive frames are seen by the two eyes in alternation. A small stationary light serves as a reference point.

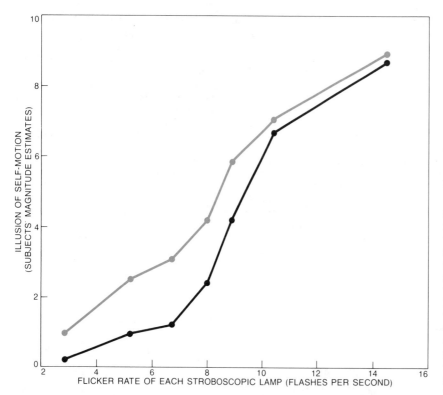

SENSATION OF VECTION is greater if the lamps are out of phase (*color*) than it is if the lamps are in phase (*black*), showing that the brain process responsible for vection can "see" a movie created by stimulating the eyes in alternation. It is thus a binocular process. The data in the chart were collected by asking six subjects to assign ratings in which 10 signified the most compelling illusion of bodily motion whereas zero signified the absence of such an illusion.

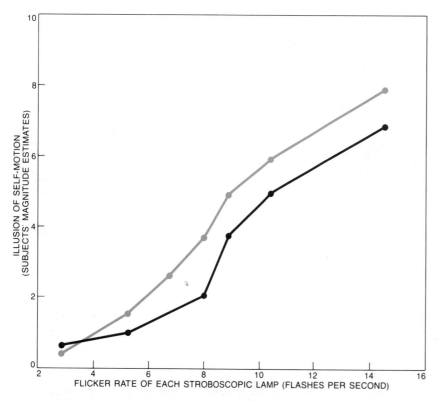

RATINGS BY STEREOBLIND SUBJECTS show that they too have a greater sensation of vection if the lamps are out of phase. People who are stereoblind lack the binocular visual process that compares the images from the eyes to aid in the perception of three-dimensional depth. Hence the process responsible for vection must be a different binocular process. The data in the chart were collected from four stereoblind subjects, who rated their sensations.

Suppose a subject looks at the chevron with only his right eye open and then manipulates the adjustable pattern with only his left eye open. The left eye never sees the chevron, yet an aftereffect is detected. In short, there is interocular transfer. It is evidence for a binocular process but not a purely binocular one. After all, the process was activated when the right eye was exposed to the chevron and it was activated when the left eye was tested with the adjustable pattern. Apparently it can respond to either the left eye or the right.

As it happens, the aftereffect is smaller when it is tested with the eye that was not exposed to the chevron than it is when it is tested with the eye that was exposed. Only 70 to 80 percent of the aftereffect transfers. Randolph Blake and his colleagues at Northwestern University conclude from this finding that at least two processes are involved when the tilt aftereffect is tested with one eye. One of them is the binocular process; the other one is monocular. Thus the exposure of the right eye to the chevron activates both the binocular process and the right eye's monocular process. The testing of the right eye activates both of them again. The result is a strong tilt aftereffect. Suppose the left eye is tested. The binocular process, which was exposed to the stimulus, becomes active again. The left eye's monocular process also becomes active, but it never "saw" the chevron. Its output dilutes the magnitude of the aftereffect.

By means, then, of the tilt aftereffect Blake demonstrated the existence of both monocular and binocular processes. Held and I exploited the aftereffect to show that a purely binocular process exists as well. We had subjects look at the chevron with each eye in alternation: one minute with the left eye, one minute with the right eye, one minute with the left eye again and one minute with the right eye again. When we measured the aftereffect, we had them keep either the left eye open, the right eye open or both eyes open.

We reasoned that the alternating monocular viewing of the stimulus would expose every visual process that gets input from the left eye, every process that gets input from the right eye and every process that gets input from either eye. If these were the only visual processes, they would constitute the entire visual system. Hence it would make no difference whether the subject had one eye open or both eyes open when he manipulated the adjustable pattern; the tilt aftereffect would be the same. If, however, there were a visual process that is active only when the left eye and the right eye are stimulated simultaneously, the results would be different. The alternating monocular viewing of the stimulus would leave this process unexposed, but then if both eyes were opened

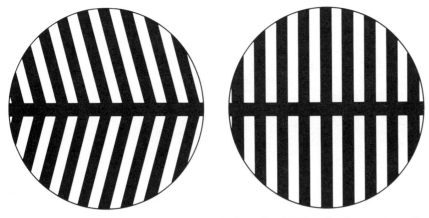

TILT AFTEREFFECT is an illusion that serves the study of hidden visual processes on the pathways leading to visual perception. To experience the illusion let your eyes scan back and forth along the horizontal black bar crossing the chevron at the left side of the illustration. You should then find that the two halves of the pattern at the right are briefly not colinear. The tilt aftereffect is measured by making the pattern at the right adjustable and asking subjects to adjust it so that it seems to be colinear immediately after they have stared at the chevron.

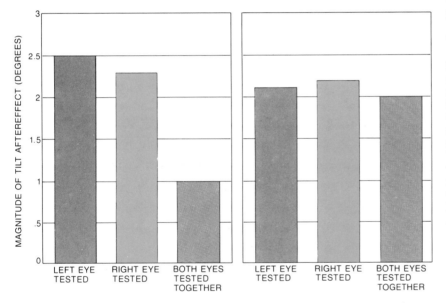

PURELY BINOCULAR PROCESS is revealed by comparing the results of two experiments that employ the tilt aftereffect. In one of the experiments (*left*) subjects stared at the chevron with each eye open in alternation; thus the stimulus was available to every visual process that gets input from one eye and every process that gets input from either eye. On the other hand, the stimulus was unavailable to a purely binocular process: one that gets input only from both eyes. The subjects then manipulated the adjustable pattern with one eye or with both eyes open. The binocular aftereffect proved to be less than the monocular aftereffect. The second experiment (*right*) differed only in that the subjects stared at the chevron with both eyes open. The binocular aftereffect now proved to equal the monocular aftereffect. Evidently the binocular viewing of the stimulus in the second experiment exposed the purely binocular process.

for the test of the aftereffect, the process would be activated, and it would dilute the aftereffect.

That is in fact what we found. The magnitude of the aftereffect was much less with both eyes open than it was with one eye closed. In a further experiment we had subjects look at the chevron with both eyes open. We expected this would expose every visual process, and we were right: the aftereffect was now much the same whether the subjects had both eyes open or one eye open when they manipulated the adjustable pattern.

In both experiments the left eye and the right eye were both exposed to the chevron. The only difference is that in the first experiment our subjects never saw the chevron with both eyes open at the same time. In the second experiment they did. A process was left unexposed by the first experiment and then was exposed in the second. That process must "see" only with both eyes. It is a purely binocular process.

What could a purely binocular process do in assistance of vision? In order to perceive three-dimensional depth the visual system seeks matches and slight mismatches between features in the images in each eye. The purely binocular process could serve in such a search. Visual perception cannot, however, be based on the output of a purely binocular process alone. If it were, all the unmatched parts of the two retinal images would vanish. In fact what we cannot see by means of a purely binocular process we can see by means of a monocular process or a process that responds to either eye.

From ancient times people have spoken of five senses. It is becoming ever clearer, however, that five is much too small a number. Senses such as touch seem to be divided into a variety of submodalities; the visual system is also divisible. Perhaps vision is best regarded not as a single sense but as a set of systems, each one a sense in its own right. It is likely that the full range of human visual senses remains to be discovered. The senses are like an old and crowded attic in that one finds the unexpected in each new corner one explores.

III

IN THE MIND'S EYE

III IN THE MIND'S EYE

INTRODUCTION

Visual perception is a creation of the brain. It is based on the input extracted from the retinal image, but what is seen in "the mind's eye" goes far beyond what is present in the input. The brain uses information it has extracted previously as the basis for educated guesses—perceptual inferences about the state of the outside world. Usually those guesses are correct and useful. On the basis of, let us say, a change in color and texture, we can conclude that there is a cat on the rug. On the basis of a continuous increase in size, we can infer that a car is coming towards us. Sometimes the inferences are wrong. The result is an illusion—we see something that is not there.

Illusions are of great use in the study of perception because, in examining the failures of the visual system, we may be able to determine the rules that govern its normal behavior. A visual illusion may literally be the exception that proves the rule.

This point is illustrated by the Kanizsa and Gillam articles. Edges are defined by differences in color or luminance between two areas, but in the real world, those differences may disappear for some distance along the boundary between two surfaces. Imagine, for example, a small piece of white paper lying on this page. It would be detected easily even though a change in luminance would only be measurable at the spots where a letter was partially covered by the paper. The rest of the contour would be "filled in" perceptually by the subjective contour mechanism discussed by Kanizsa. Kanizsa argues that this completion occurs fairly late in visual processing and his view has recently received some interesting physiological support. Cells up to and including those in the primary visual cortex (see the Hubel and Wiesel article) do not respond to subjective edges, but only to real ones. However, Peterhans, von der Heydt, and Bamgartner in Zurich have recently found cells at the next stage of visual processing that will respond to such edges.

Gillam deals with some of the most familiar misperceptions, the geometrical illusions. She regards them as mistakes made by the mechanisms that create a three-dimensional world out of a two-dimensional image. It is not that we see the illusory figures as three-dimensional, but rather that depth-finding processes operating on the two-dimensional image can distort the apparent size and shape of contours.

The illusions that concern Hoffman are those involving perceptual ambiguity. Most visual input is ambiguous. The majority of the time, however, the visual system quickly reaches an unambiguous interpretation of the stimulus. Consider again the piece of paper lying on the page in front of you. On the basis of the input alone, it could be that there is a hole in the page through which you can see a white surface. The heart of Hoffman's article is that the visual system has access to information that eliminates such inaccuracies as perceptual possibilities. Inferences based on regularities in the world constrain perception, and constraints usually reduce the ambiguities to a single percept. In some cases, two possibilities may remain, and the result is an ambiguous figure.

Sometimes what is seen by the mind's eye is not based directly on input. Certain forms of perception are generated from within. For example, suppose you were asked about the number of windows in your parents' home. To answer, you would probably take a mental walking tour, counting windows from imagined room to imagined room. If asked how to get a kitchen table out one of those windows, you would probably conjure up an image of the table and mentally rotate it until it "fits." Cooper and Shepard have brought this ability to generate and manipulate mental images into the lab, where they have found that it behaves in a very lawful manner. Even though mental images are not tied to visual input, many of the rules that govern perception also limit the behavior of these images.

Finally, there are hallucinations, perceptions generated from within the brain not by an act of will, but by abnormal neural activity. Siegel finds that, for all their bizarre qualities, hallucinations are also governed by perceptual rules. For example, some hallucinations seem to result from abnormal stimulation of visual cortex. The perception is of little lines or blobs, some with color, some with motion. It is as though the visual system were extracting features from a nonexistent stimulus. The features are smaller in the center of the pattern, just as visual resolution is finer at the point of fixation. The pattern of small central features growing larger towards the edge of the field is often described as a tunnel.

So, even when the input is abnormal, the visual system attempts to apply its rules of inference. It is important to realize that most of this takes place automatically, without conscious intervention or thought. The unusual occurrences in perception, the illusions and hallucinations, reveal the complex machinery that supports the seemingly effortless act of normal vision.

8

Subjective Contours

by Gaetano Kanizsa
April 1976

*Certain combinations of incomplete figures give rise to clearly
visible contours even when the contours do not actually exist.
It appears that such contours are supplied by the visual

I f we examine the conditions that give rise to visible contours, we usually find that a contour is perceived when there is a jump in the stimulation between adjacent areas. The jump may be due to a difference in brightness or a difference in color. There are conditions, however, that cause us to perceive contours in visual areas that are completely homogeneous. For example, in the illustration below the solid triangles in the center of each figure appear to have well-defined contours, but close examination of the contours where they cross an open area reveals that they have no physical basis. If you fix your gaze on one of these contours, it disappears, yet if you direct your gaze to the entire figure, the contours appear to be real.

The phenomenon of contours that appear in the absence of physical gradients has aroused considerable interest among psychologists on both the experimental and the theoretical level. A number of variants of the effect have been discovered, and several explanations have been proposed for it. Here I shall describe some of the more interesting properties of the effect and examine some of the attempted explanations.

First, however, let us consider a related visual phenomenon: the phenomenon of virtual lines.

When we view three dots that are equidistant from one another and are not in a straight line, the visual system spontaneously organizes the dots into a triangle. In addition the three dots appear to be connected by three straight lines. These lines are called virtual, and although they are not actually seen, they are a real presence in our visual experience. They are far more compelling than other connecting lines that can be imagined. For example, the three dots

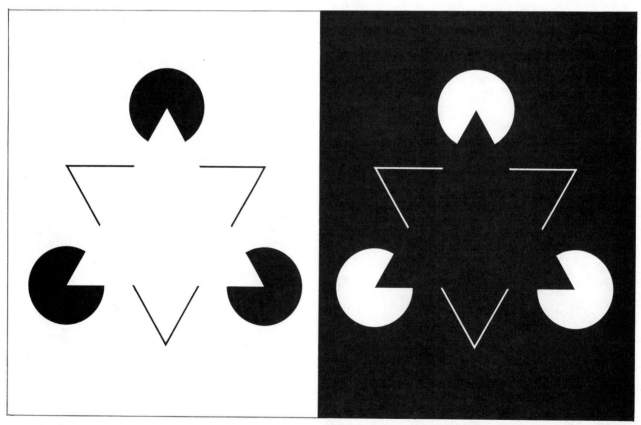

TWO SUBJECTIVE TRIANGLES, one whiter than white and the other blacker than black, appear to have distinct contours, but when the contours are examined closely, they disappear. The contours are subjective and have no physical reality. The region bounded by the subjective contours appears to be more intense than the background even though the color of the inner and the outer regions is identical.

could just as readily be points on a circle, but the curved connecting lines of the circle are more difficult to "see" than the straight lines of the triangle.

Because virtual lines are only phenomenally present and do not have a sensory modality, one may speak of them as being "amodal." Another kind of amodal contour is found in partially hidden figures [*see top illustration at right*]. Consider a black rectangle that has a gray ring behind it and a colored ring in front of it. Although the missing contours of the rectangle are not actually seen, they nonetheless have a strong phenomenal presence. If the two rings in the illustration are now made black, a new effect results. Both black rings complete themselves behind the black rectangle in an amodal manner, but the contours of the rectangle are visible in their entirety. Even in the homogeneous black regions where the rings overlap, the contours of the rectangle are visible. In other words, the contours have acquired a visual modality.

This "modal" presence is also found in the contours of the central triangles in the illustration on the opposite page. Since those contours appear in the absence of the gradients that normally produce modal, or visible, contours, the situation is clearly anomalous. For that reason I prefer to call such contours anomalous contours. In order to emphasize the fact that the contours have no physical basis over most of their length, other investigators have called them subjective contours. They are also known as illusory contours. Whatever term is used, the phenomenon is the same.

W hat factors are involved in the formation of subjective contours? Analysis of many examples of the phenomenon yields the following common characteristics. First, the region that is bounded by the subjective contours appears to be brighter than the background, even though the visual stimulation provided by both regions is exactly the same. Second, the region within the subjective contours appears as an opaque surface that is superposed on the other figures in the illustration.

The subjective contours we have considered up to this point have all been straight lines. Is it possible to create curved subjective contours? As the middle and bottom illustrations at the right demonstrate, there are a variety of ways for generating such subjective contours. Indeed, even amorphous subjective figures can be created.

The strength of the phenomenon of subjective contours can be measured in part by determining the resistance such contours show to interference by real lines. When a real line intersects a subjective contour, the contour in that region disappears, indicating that it has a relatively low degree of resistance to interference. On the other hand, the opaque subjective surface displays surprising resistance: it appears to pass under lines that intersect it [*see top illustration on page 85*]. The subjective

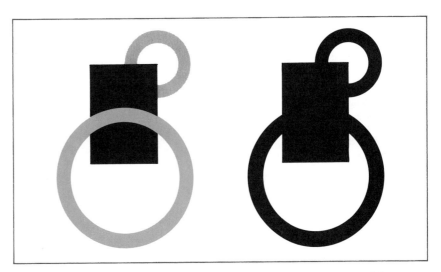

AMODAL AND MODAL CONTOURS are found in overlapping figures. Amodal contours are not actually seen, but they have a strong phenomenal presence. For example, the missing contours of the black rectangle complete themselves behind the colored ring in an amodal manner. Modal contours, on the other hand, appear to be visible. For example, the contours of the rectangle at the right are visible even in the regions where they overlap the black rings.

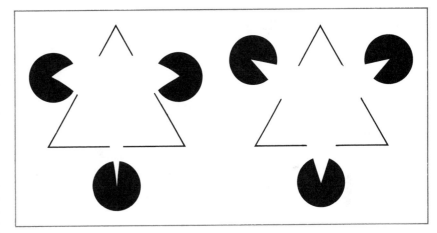

CURVED SUBJECTIVE CONTOURS are created by sectors with curved angles (*left*). Sectors with straight angles can create curved contours if angles are not aligned with one another.

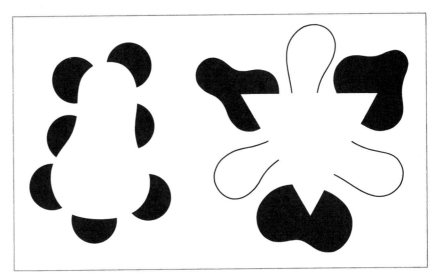

GEOMETRIC REGULARITY is not a necessary condition for the formation of subjective surfaces and contours. Amorphous shapes are possible and irregular figures can generate contours.

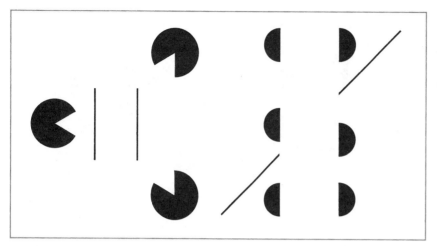

OPTICAL ILLUSIONS show that subjective contours have the same functional effects as real contours. In the Ponzo illusion (*left*), although both vertical lines are the same length, the effect of the subjective triangle is to make the line at the left appear to be longer. In the Poggendorf illusion the subjective surface gives rise to an apparent displacement of the slanted line.

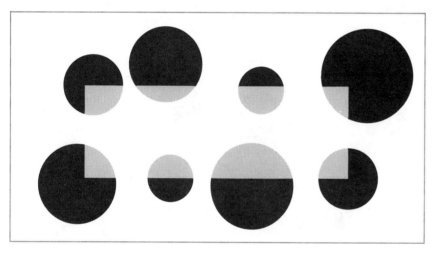

TRANSPARENT SUBJECTIVE SURFACES, as well as opaque ones, can be produced. The transparent surface, with clearly visible contours, seems to lie in a plane in front of black disks.

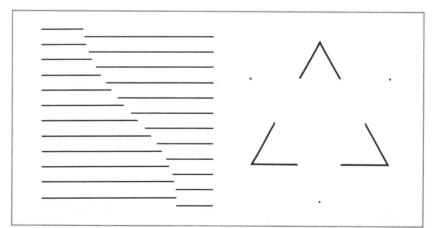

CONTOUR-DETECTOR HYPOTHESIS states that subjective contours are generated by partial activation of contour detectors in the visual system by short line segments in the stimulus. Subjective contours, however, can have an orientation completely different from that of the line segments (*left*). Furthermore, line segments are not necessary for generation of subjective contours (*right*). Curved subjective contour formed by line segments also demonstrates that differences in brightness due to contrast are not needed for formation of subjective contours.

surface also displays strong resistance to interference within its borders. If large dark spots are placed inside the borders, the spots do not become part of the background but rather appear to be on the subjective surface. What happens when the background, instead of being homogeneous, has a texture? It turns out that a texture does not impede the formation of subjective contours or surfaces.

A number of optical illusions are produced by the reciprocal action between lines and surfaces. These optical illusions offer an opportunity to ascertain whether subjective contours and shapes have the same functional effects as objective, or real, contours and shapes. In many instances subjective contours and shapes are able to duplicate the illusion created by objective ones. As the top illustration at the left demonstrates, subjective contours and surfaces will interact with physically real lines to give rise to familiar optical illusions.

As we have seen, one of the characteristics of subjective surfaces is that they appear to be superposed on the other figures in the illustration. We have also seen that the subjective surface appears to be opaque. It is not difficult, however, to produce transparent subjective surfaces with distinct subjective contours [*see middle illustration at left*].

In most of the situations we have been examining the subjective surface appears to be brighter than the background, even though the two regions are identical in brightness and color. It is possible that the brightness of the subjective surface is due to contrast enhancement. Such enhancement is generally found when a light surface is adjacent to one dark surface or more. The intensity of the effect depends on the extent of the dark surface. Although the brightness-contrast effect may play a role in creating subjective surfaces, it is not a necessary condition for the formation of such surfaces or contours. This is readily demonstrated in the middle illustration on the opposite page, where a substantial reduction in the amount of black does not diminish the effect. A decisive item of evidence that contrast is not necessary for the formation of a subjective contour is presented in the figure at the left in the bottom illustration at the left. In this figure there are no differences in brightness that could be attributed to contrast, yet a curved subjective contour between the line segments is clearly visible.

It has been suggested by some investigators that subjective contours can be explained in terms of the partial activation of contour-detector cells in the visual system. According to this hypothesis, the short line segments in the visual stimulus activate some of the contour detectors, and signals from the activated detectors are interpreted as being a stimulus from a continuous line. The hypothesis does not stand up to careful examination, however. In many cases a subjective contour does not continue in the same direction as the stimulus line seg-

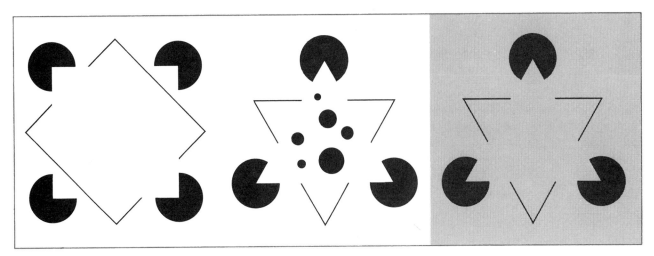

RESISTANCE TO INTERFERENCE is a measure of the perceptual strength of subjective surfaces. A subjective surface appears to pass under lines that intersect with it (*left*), but subjective contours are destroyed by the line. Spots inside the borders of the subjective surface become part of it (*middle*). The formation of subjective contours or surfaces is not impeded by the presence of a texture (*right*).

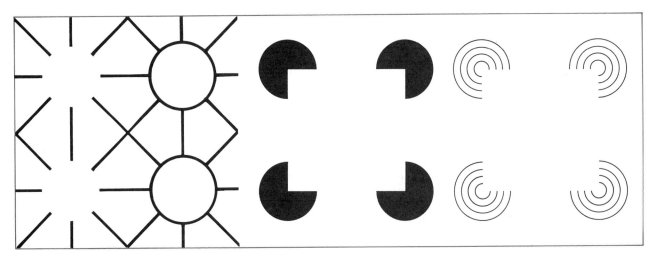

ENHANCED BRIGHTNESS of subjective surfaces is not due to contrast. If contrast were a primary condition of the effect, the black-ringed circles should appear to be brighter than the subjective circles (*left*). Reducing amount of black does not diminish the effect (*right*).

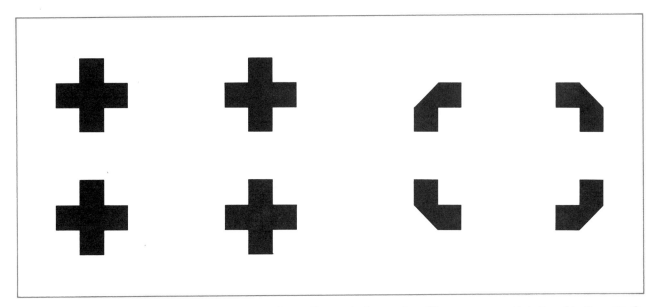

COMPLETE FIGURES do not generate subjective surfaces. Although crosses provide outlines of a rectangle, the rectangle is not perceived as a surface. When crosses are cut in half, a subjective rectangle is perceived and the half crosses are now seen as mutilated hexagons.

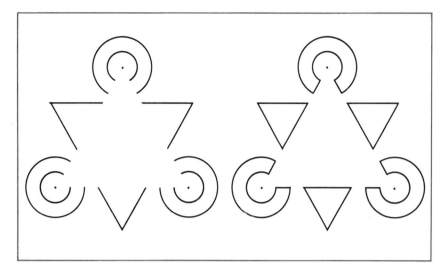

FIGURES WITH OPEN BORDERS appear to be incomplete. In order to complete the figures the visual system superposes an opaque surface that fills the gaps in the figures. Because the surface must have borders the necessary contours are also supplied by the visual system. If borders of figures are closed, there is no further need for completion and contours disappear.

ments. Moreover, line segments are not necessary for the generation of subjective contours. In some instances the line segments can be replaced by dots and subjective contours will still be perceived [*see figure at right in bottom illustration on page 84*].

There is one condition, I have found, that is always present in the formation of subjective contours. That condition is the presence in the visual field of certain elements that are incomplete, which on completion are transformed into simpler stable and regular figures. For example, it could be said that the figure at the left in the illustration on page 48 consists of three black sectors and three angles. Each of these figural elements is incomplete in some way. Most observers, however, report that they see a white triangle covering three black disks and another triangle with a black border. This perceptual organization has obvious advantages from the standpoint of simplicity and stability. The three angles become a

triangle, a stabler and more balanced figure. The three circular sectors acquire completeness and regularity by becoming disks. In order for this perceptual organization to materialize, however, the white area in the center must be seen as an opaque triangle that is superposed on the other figures. And since the triangle must have a border, the necessary contours are supplied by the visual system. The contours are therefore the result of perceiving a surface and not vice versa. The subjective surface in turn is generated by the tendency of the visual system to complete certain figural elements.

If these assertions are correct, we should be able to demonstrate that subjective contours and shapes will not be perceived when the visual field does not contain incomplete figural elements. Since figures with open borders tend to appear incomplete, it is not difficult to create subjective contours with them. If we close the borders on these figures and make no other changes, the subjec-

tive contours disappear [*see top illustration on this page*].

The following, I believe, offers further confirmation of the completion hypothesis. At the left in the bottom illustration on the preceding page there are four black crosses on a white field. In spite of the fact that the crosses provide the outlines of a rectangle in the central region, we do not perceive the rectangle as a subjective surface. The reason is that the crosses are balanced and self-sufficient figures and do not require completion. When the crosses are cut in half, however, a subjective surface appears in the central area. The half crosses are in this case more likely to be seen as mutilated hexagons.

We have seen that irregularly shaped subjective figures can be produced. In most of my examples the incomplete figures I have used to create subjective contours have been regular and symmetrical. Although geometric figures may enhance the effect, however, they are by no means necessary [*see bottom illustration on page 83*].

Finally, is it possible to generate subjective contours that meet and form a subjective angle? Paolo Sambin of the University of Padua found that an incomplete cross gives rise to such an effect [*see bottom illustration on this page*]. According to Sambin, the rectangular shape of the subjective surface that is perceived is produced by the resistance of the arms of the cross to invasion by the subjective surface. Without such resistance the subjective contour would assume the shape of a circle. The validity of his hypothesis can be demonstrated by narrowing the arms of the cross to the point where the invasion of the internal area is minimal. Under those conditions the subjective surface that is perceived has the form of a circle.

Another example of contour perception in the absence of brightness gradients is found in the random-dot stereograms created by Bela Julesz of Bell Laboratories. These stereograms do not reveal any contours when they are viewed monocularly, but when they are viewed with a stereoscope, they combine to form three-dimensional shapes and contours. Stanley Coren of the New School for Social Research has advanced the hypothesis that the perceptual mechanism giving rise to subjective contours and shapes is the same as the mechanism giving rise to three-dimensional depth perception.

Since the formation of subjective contours is usually connected with the generation of surfaces and their stratification, or apparent layering, the line of reasoning proposed by Coren may be valid. On the other hand, in all the cases that we have examined stratification depends on the completion of some figural elements. When there is no need for completion, stratification does not occur and there are no subjective contours. Once more the primary factor seems to be the tendency to completion. Stratification seems to arise as a function of this completion.

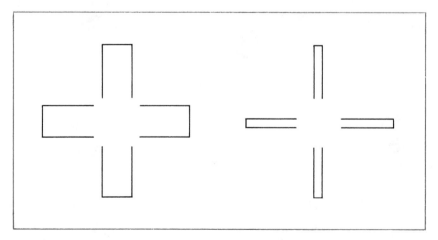

INCOMPLETE CROSS (*left*) gives rise to the unusual phenomenon of subjective angles. The angles are formed by the contours of the subjective square that covers central portion of the cross. Rectangular shape of the subjective surface is attributed to the resistance of arms of cross to invasion by the surface. If arms of cross are narrowed, circular subjective surface results.

9

Geometrical Illusions

by Barbara Gillam
January 1980

*In these classic figures of psychology lines appear different
from the way they really are. The effects appear to be related
to clues to the size of objects in the three-dimensional world*

Geometrical illusions are line figures in which the length, orientation, curvature or direction of lines is wrongly perceived. For example, in certain figures two lines of equal length appear to differ in length. Why does this happen? In normal three-dimensional viewing two lines of unequal length at different distances from the observer can cast on the retina images of equal size, but the lines are not perceived as being equal because the visual system takes into account the fact that they lie at different distances. The lines appear to have the lengths they actually have in the three-dimensional world because the perceptual mechanism known as size constancy seems to compensate for the difference in distance by making the far line appear to be larger and the near line appear to be smaller. It has been suggested that size constancy is responsible for geometrical illusions. In other words, if the visual system processed the lines of a geometric figure as if they were at different distances, then the result would be an illusion.

Attractive as this explanation of illusions may be, it is not correct because in most illusory line figures there is no depth, either real or apparent. It has nonetheless seemed to several investigators, including me, that some process contributing to accurate perceptions of the three-dimensional world might give rise to illusions in two-dimensional figures. My own finding is that geometrical illusions depend not on apparent depth but on clues to the scale and size of objects in the visible world, clues such as linear perspective and foreshortening. I shall be returning to this distinction between apparent depth and perspective clues in somewhat greater detail.

Most of the more than 200 geometric illusions that have been recorded by investigators were discovered in the second half of the 19th century. Some of the best-known illusions are shown in the illustration on the opposite page. In the Müller-Lyer figure the two lines, one with outward-pointing arrowheads at the ends and the other with inward-pointing arrowheads, are actually the same length. In the Ponzo figure the horizontal lines are also the same length. In both the Zöllner and Lipps figures the oblique lines are parallel. In the Titchener figure the two inner circles are the same size. In the Delboeuf figure the outer circle on the left is the same size as the inner circle on the right. In the Poggendorff figure the oblique lines are collinear. In the upside-down *T* the horizontal and vertical lines are the same length. And in the Judd figure the dot is at the middle of the horizontal line.

Each of these illusions has traditionally been thought to consist of two parts: an "inducing" component that does the distorting and a "test" component that is distorted. For example, in the Müller-Lyer figure the arrowheads are the inducing component and the horizontal lines are the test component, and in the Poggendorff figure the parallel lines are the inducing component and the oblique lines are the test component. This division can, however, oversimplify what is going on. The distortion of the test component is sometimes only the most obvious manifestation of a host of misperceptions that involve the inducing component as well.

In the 100 years that geometrical illusions have been studied many different explanations for them have been advanced. The most compelling of these explanations agree on three fundamental points. First, the illusions are not conceptual but perceptual; knowing that a particular effect is illusory does not diminish the strength of the illusion, although most of the illusions are drastically reduced when the figure is viewed repeatedly over a short period of time. Second, the illusions do not originate in the retina; they emerge at almost full strength when the inducing component is presented to one eye and the test component is presented to the other, and so they must originate at a point in the visual system beyond the lateral geniculate nucleus of the brain, where the inputs from the two eyes first come together. Third, illusions do not result from the movements of the eye; experiments show that the illusions, usually of full magnitude, emerge when a figure is exposed too briefly for the eye to scan it or when the retinal image of the figure is artificially stabilized by a special apparatus that causes the image to remain still on the retina even as the eye moves back and forth.

Explanations of illusions fall into four main categories: classification theories, activity theories, physiological theories and functional theories. The theories are not necessarily mutually exclusive; in some cases they might emphasize different aspects of the same process. The first of these categories is the least ambitious. The classification theories point to common properties among a variety of illusory figures. What the figures have in common suggests the presence of an underlying perceptual process. Neither the mechanism nor the function of such a process is addressed by the classification theories. The illusions are attributed to contrast when they are characterized by a perceptual exaggeration of the degree to which the test component differs from the inducing component in a prevailing quality such as size or orientation. The Titchener illusion is an example of size contrast, whereas the Zöllner illusion is one of orientation contrast, or more specifically of angle contrast.

The illusions are attributed to assimilation or confusion when they are characterized by a perceptual underestimation of the degree to which the test component differs from the inducing component. In other words, the test element is distorted in the same direction as a prevailing quality of the inducing element. The Müller-Lyer illusion is an example of size or position assimilation because the horizontal lines are lengthened in the direction of the arrowheads. The Lipps illusion is an example of orientation assimilation because the orientation of each parallel line is perceptually shifted toward the orientation of its neighbors. A single illusion can incorporate both contrast and assimilation. In the Ponzo illusion the apparent length of the upper line is distorted toward the surround (assimilation), whereas the apparent length of the lower line is distorted away from the surround (contrast).

This classification scheme has done little more than help to bring order to the large number of illusions. It does suggest, however, that the processes could have something in common with those of brightness perception, which exhibits both contrast and assimilation with respect to the brightness of neighboring areas in a scene. Apart from the classification scheme's lack of explanatory power, it is limited by the fact that it does not apply to some important illusions, for example the Poggendorff figure and the upside-down *T*. Moreover, the lines that are assimilated in the Lipps figure are well within the orientation range of the lines that show contrast in the Zöllner figure.

The activity and physiological theories go beyond mere classification by asserting that illusions are incidental side effects or errors of normal visual perception. Activity theories attribute illusions to the responses an individual has to certain stimuli or prepares to have to them. The efferent-readiness theory, proposed by Leon Festinger of the New School for Social Research, maintains that illusions develop because of the way the eye "gets ready" for saccadic movements. (As I have mentioned, experimental evidence rules out the eye movements themselves playing a role in the illusions, but that evidence does not rule out the possibility that the visual system's preparations for eye movements do play such a role.) According to this theory, people tend to look not at the entire figure but at the part of the figure that optimizes the number of details seen with high acuity. Festinger and his co-workers have found that when people try to fixate on the ends of a Müller-Lyer figure, they actually fixate within the arrowheads. According to Festinger, that has the effect of lengthening the line with the inward-pointing arrowheads and shortening the line with the outward-pointing ones.

It is known that the decrease in the strength of an illusion that comes with repeated exposure is accompanied by an increase in the accuracy of eye movements, but this correlation does not indicate whether or not the eye movements cause the illusions. Many other motor responses, such as directing a pointer at the illusion, might provide information about the perceptual error and thereby help to reduce the illusion in the same way that eye movements do. Inasmuch as the illusion would not be attributed to the intention to direct a pointer, it would be premature in the absence of other evidence to attribute the illusion to preparations for saccadic eye movements. Moreover, it is difficult to understand why inaccurate eye movements in the presence of angle and line intersections would not have been eliminated in the normal environment where such intersections are frequently encountered.

The physiological theories attribute illusions to the "hardware" of the visual system. Many of these theories are based on lateral inhibition, a neural process that serves to restrict the stimuli that can fire a cell in the visual cortex of the brain. According to these theories, the perceived orientation of a line is determined by the peak activity of orientation-detecting cells in the visual cortex, each of which is activated by line stimuli of a particular range of orientations. The introduction of a second line of a different but similar orientation gives rise to a somewhat different distribution of activity among the orientation-detecting cells, activity that either facilitates or inhibits the activity generated by the first line, thereby shifting the apparent orientation. On this view facilitation, which would result from very similar

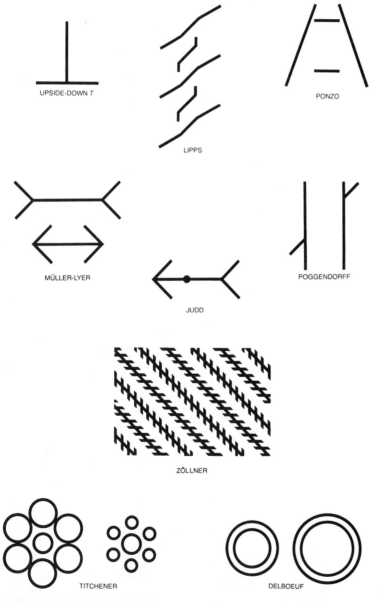

NINE GEOMETRICAL ILLUSIONS are presented on the opposite page. In the upside-down-*T* figure the vertical line and the horizontal line are the same length. In the Lipps figure the oblique lines in the middle are parallel. In both the Ponzo figure and the Müller-Lyer figure the horizontal lines are equal in length. In the Judd figure the dot is at the midpoint of the horizontal line. In the Poggendorff figure the oblique lines are collinear. In the Zöllner figure the oblique lines are parallel. In the Titchener figure the two inner circles are the same size. In the Delboeuf figure the outer circle on the left is the same size as the inner circle on the right.

lines, would cause assimilation in the illusory figure, and inhibition, which would result from less similar lines, would cause contrast. The same view is supported by the experiments of Colin Blakemore and his co-workers at the University of Cambridge. To explain size illusions a similar physiological theory has been proposed that is based on size-detecting cells in the visual cortex.

Physiological theories based on lateral inhibition are best able to handle angle-contrast illusions with multiple inducing lines, for example the Zöllner illusion, which exhibits assimilation at extremely small angles and contrast at larger angles. George Wallace and his co-workers at the University of Reading have found that the Zöllner illusion is enhanced by changes that should promote lateral inhibition, such as increasing either the brightness contrast or the number of inducing lines.

Most angle-contrast illusions persist when the test line is replaced by a set of dots or by a moving dot. Physiological theories based on lateral inhibition cannot explain this phenomenon because there is no actual test line to be inhibited. That may not be a problem, however, because little work has been done on whether the orientation-detecting cells might in fact respond selectively not only to a line but also to a row of dots or a moving dot.

Physiological theories based on lateral inhibition fall short for the simplest illusions involving angles. For example, in the Poggendorff figure the acute angles, which should show the greatest effect of lateral inhibition, contribute nothing to the illusion [see top illustration on next page]. Another exception is the Müller-Lyer illusion, which no physiological theory has been able to explain. A comparison of the horizontal lines of the Müller-Lyer figure with a line lacking arrowheads reveals that the inward-pointing-arrowhead configuration (obtuse angles) contributes two or three times as much to the total illusion as the outward-pointing-arrowhead configuration (acute angles). No plausible arrangement of orientation-detecting cells could give rise to such lopsided contributions.

Another physiological theory, filter theory, is based on neural channels in the visual cortex that seem to be tuned not to line stimuli but to particular spatial frequencies of sinusoidal modulations of light, the spatial frequency being the number of modulations per unit of visual angle. Mathematicians have proved that any waveform, no matter how complicated, can be expressed as the sum of simple sinusoidal waveforms. In 1968 Fergus W. Campbell and John G. Robson of the University of Cambridge proposed that the visual system processes a waveform of light by

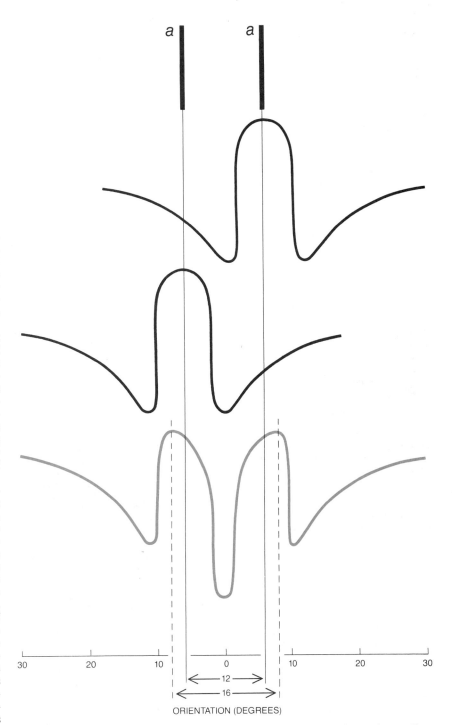

VISUAL RESPONSE TO LINE STIMULI is shown in a highly schematic way for two lines (a) that differ in orientation by 12 degrees. Below each line is the distribution of orientation-detecting cells of the visual cortex that the line activates. The colored distribution shows what might happen if the two lines were presented simultaneously to the visual system. The sum of the individual distributions gives rise to the colored distribution in which the peaks of activity are slightly displaced from each other. This illustration is based on the findings of Colin Blakemore, Roger H. S. Carpenter and their colleagues at the University of Cambridge.

breaking it down into its sinusoidal components. Since then much psychophysical and physiological evidence has accumulated in support of this proposal, and it is now a cornerstone of visual theory.

Arthur Ginsberg of the U.S. Air Force attributes illusions to the responses of the neural channels that are tuned to low spatial frequencies. He has broken down the images of certain illusory figures into sinusoidal waveforms of different frequencies and amplitudes, eliminated the high-frequency waveforms and added back together the low-frequency ones. With the high-frequency waveforms filtered out the reconstruct-

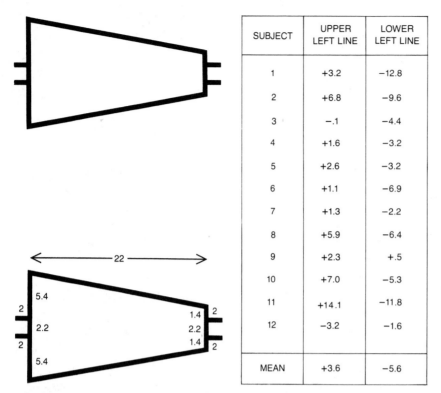

SUBJECT	UPPER LEFT LINE	LOWER LEFT LINE
1	+3.2	−12.8
2	+6.8	−9.6
3	−.1	−4.4
4	+1.6	−3.2
5	+2.6	−3.2
6	+1.1	−6.9
7	+1.3	−2.2
8	+5.9	−6.4
9	+2.3	+.5
10	+7.0	−5.3
11	+14.1	−11.8
12	−3.2	−1.6
MEAN	+3.6	−5.6

VARIATION OF THE PONZO ILLUSION at the top left consists of collinear line segments that seem to be displaced. The line at the upper right appears to be too high and the line at the lower right appears to be too low for them to be aligned with their counterparts at the left. The author asked 12 subjects to indicate how much each line at the left should be adjusted so that it would be collinear with the corresponding line at the right. For the figure at the bottom left with dimensions in centimeters the subjects' adjustments are tabulated in millimeters at the right. In the normal Ponzo illusion in the illustration on page 88 the apparent length of the upper line is distorted toward the surround (the distortion called assimilation), whereas the apparent length of the lower line is distorted away from the surround (the distortion called contrast). Yet there is more to the illusion. The figure at the top left shows that the Ponzo configuration affects not only length of lines placed in it but also alignment of lines attached to its ends.

ed image turns out to have properties that correspond to perceived distortions of the original figure. For example, in the reconstructed image of the outward-pointing-arrowhead configuration of the Müller-Lyer illusion the arrowheads and the shaft have merged to form a short blurred shaft, and in the reconstructed image of the inward-pointing-arrowhead configuration the arrowheads and the shaft have merged to form a long blurred shaft. The respective shortening and lengthening of the shaft is of course the substance of the illusion.

Ingenious as Ginsberg's work may be, there is little reason to believe that in arriving at size judgments the visual system filters out the information provided by high-frequency waveforms. It would be odd (although not impossible) if the visual system judged the apparent size of a distinct line by the responses of neural channels in which the line was indistinctly merged with its surround, particularly because such judgments would lead to gross perceptual errors.

A major drawback of both activity theories and physiological theories is that they cannot account for the de-

creases in the strength of illusions. The fact that by repeated exposure illusions can diminish almost to zero for as long as a period of days does not support theories that posit immutable physiological mechanisms. Only functional theories, which treat illusions not as errors but as essential processes of the visual system, begin to deal adequately with decreases in the strength of illusions.

Over the past century several investigators, including the 19th-century psychologist Armand Thiéry, Richard L. Gregory of the University of Bristol and Reinhardt Tausch of the University of Marburg, have shown that most illusory figures can be found in two-dimensional representations of three-dimensional scenes. What are called distortions or illusions in sketchy drawings promote accurate perception in the normal three-dimensional world and increase the realism of a picture. Consider the bottom illustration at the left. One guitar looks longer than the other (the Ponzo illusion), the rear edge of the carpet looks shorter than its front-to-back dimension (the upside-down *T*), the molding looks too high to be collinear with the base-

board (the Poggendorff illusion) and the front edge of the carpet looks shorter than the bottom edge of the back wall (the Müller-Lyer illusion with half of each arrowhead).

Although all these percepts are distortions compared with the picture plane or the retinal image, they would not normally be called illusions because they are not surprising. They reflect characteristics of the three-dimensional world represented in the picture plane. In normal three-dimensional viewing it is quite irrelevant whether or not a baseboard is retinally collinear with a molding and whether or not the edge of a door has the same length in the retinal image as the corner of a room. Such facts about the picture plane, which depend mostly on the viewing position of the observer, are not registered.

The main function of perception is to decode the transient retinal image in order to achieve constancy: the perception of the external world in terms of its stable and intrinsic characteristics. In the illustration of the room it is clear that the "distortions" are just instances of perception doing its job. If the contextual details that are necessary for a three-dimensional impression are eliminated, however, the same perceptual responses to the same configurations seem unjustified and are called illusions. Does this mean that illusions are only constancy responses (the decoding of perspective) operating in a context that is too minimal, since it lacks apparent depth, to give the distortions meaning? This view is appealingly parsimonious, but it goes against a strong tradition in psychology that constancy responses are triggered by apparent depth.

There are a number of reasons to doubt that a depth response always underlies constancy scaling. J. J. Gibson of Cornell University has pointed out that gradients in the apparent compression of objects and textures by perspective provide information about the size and shape of objects. The size of an object can often be judged by the ratio of its width to the width of the background. Consider railroad tracks receding into the distance. Since the viewer knows that the distant railroad ties are as large as the close ones, an object spanning the rails in the distance is perceived as being the same size as an object spanning the rails in the foreground, in spite of the fact that the sizes of the objects' retinal images are quite different.

Conclusive evidence for a size-constancy process that is not secondary to perceived depth comes from my own work with backgrounds in which equivalent depths are represented by different types of perspective [*see illustrations on page 92*]. In effect I was able to separate the response to depth from the response to perspective. I investigated two kinds of background drawing. In the first kind, based on the receding oblique lines of the Ponzo figure, the horizontal dimensions are increasingly compressed toward the "far" end, or top, of the drawing (the distortion known as linear perspective). In the second drawing, based on horizontal parallel lines that get closer to one another toward the top of the drawing, the vertical dimensions are increasingly compressed (the distortion known as foreshortening).

Next I put test lines at various orientations on the two kinds of background. I found that the perceptual lengthening of lines put at the top with respect to lines put at the "near" end, or bottom, occurred only when the test lines were oriented along the compressed dimensions. There was no illusion for test lines at orientations for which the background drawing did not provide a scale of size. In other words, a linear-perspective scale does not affect the apparent length of lines along the dimension subject to foreshortening. This result constitutes compelling evidence for a perceptual mechanism promoting size constancy that is based on the scale itself and not on a depth response to the scale, which would lengthen any apparently distant lines regardless of their orientation.

This is not to deny that apparent distance can influence size perception. Experiments have demonstrated that changes in perceived size and shape accompany depth reversal in ambiguous figures. The fact that perceived size and shape can be primary responses and yet can still be influenced by apparent depth is not surprising when one considers that depth perception itself can be influenced by apparent size and shape. An example is the well-known moon illusion. When the moon is near the horizon, it looks larger than it does high in the sky. As a result when it is near the horizon, it looks closer. Under normal circumstances primary and secondary ways of judging size and distance reinforce each other. My work shows, however, that the amount of information in a line drawing needed to trigger a primary process of size scaling is less than the amount needed to trigger a process of depth scaling. Gregory has suggested that this result may be due to a perceptual conflict between the drawing's representing objects in depth and its actually being flat.

How well can a functional theory based not on apparent depth but on perspective explain illusions that do not have an interpretation as obvious in terms of perspective as the Ponzo illusion does? How does it explain the Müller-Lyer or the Poggendorff illusion? The resemblance between the Müller-Lyer figure and objects and scenes involving depth has been recognized since the 19th century. Most recently Gregory

has pointed to the similarity between the two Müller-Lyer configurations and the corner of a building seen respectively from the inside and the outside. On the other hand, Tausch and other investigators, including me, have found that the Müller-Lyer illusion is close to being the sum of the separate effects of the four individual oblique lines forming the arrowheads on the length of the horizontal line, effects that seem to be divorced from depth. Two lines that

form acute angles are perceptually shortened, whereas two that form obtuse angles are lengthened. It is the distortion of these fundamental angle relations that must be understood in order to comprehend the Müller-Lyer illusions and other illusions in which angles influence perceived line length.

Do the lengthening of lines bounded by obtuse angles and the shortening of lines bounded by acute angles promote perceptual constancy? They do.

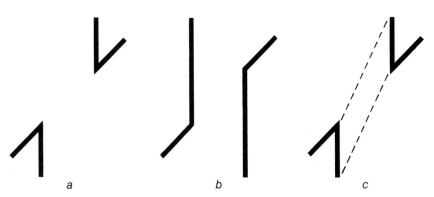

POGGENDORFF FIGURE is decomposed so that the illusory effects of the acute-angle components (a) can be distinguished from those of the obtuse-angle components (b). In a the illusion is zero or even slightly negative, the line at the right appearing to some people to be slightly lower than the one at the left. In b the illusion is strongly present. An illusion in a may be due to the visual system's processing a as if it were part of c, in which parallel lines form a receding plane. In c the line at the right is in fact lower on the receding plane than the one at left.

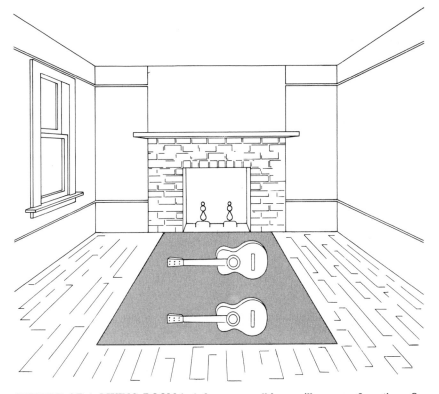

PICTURE OF A LIVING ROOM includes many well-known illusory configurations. One guitar looks longer than the other (Ponzo illusion), the rear edge of the carpet looks shorter than its front-to-back dimension (upside-down-T illusion), the molding looks too high to be collinear with the baseboard (Poggendorff illusion) and the front edge of the carpet looks shorter than the bottom edge of the back wall (Müller-Lyer illusion with half of each arrowhead).

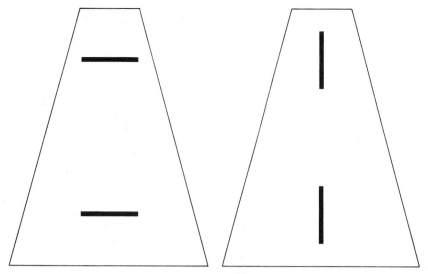

LINEAR PERSPECTIVE, the compression of horizontal dimensions toward the top of a draw-ing, is achieved by the receding oblique lines of the Ponzo figure. The horizontal test lines (*left*) are the same length, but the upper line appears to be longer because of linear perspective. There is no illusion for vertical test lines (*right*). This means that here the perception of size depends not on depth, which would increase the length of all the test lines regardless of their orientation, but on perspective, which affects only lines for which the background shows a scale of size.

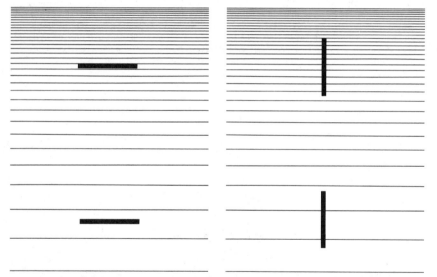

FORESHORTENING, the compression of vertical dimensions toward the top of a drawing, is achieved by parallel horizontal lines that get closer to one another toward the top of the draw-ing. The vertical test lines (*right*) are the same length, but the upper one seems longer because of foreshortening. There is no illusion for the horizontal test lines (*left*). This result confirms that the perception of size here does not depend on depth, which would lengthen horizontal lines as well as vertical ones. Perception of size seems to depend on the perspective scale of size.

An overwhelmingly large proportion of the obtuse and acute angles formed on the retina in the course of human visu-al experience are projections of right angles. A perceptual mechanism that lengthens horizontal lines bounded by obtuse angles and shortens horizontal lines bounded by acute angles would compensate for the differences in size created by perspective projection [*see top illustration on page 93*].

The illustration also shows that the

process I have described would promote size and shape constancy regardless of whether the obtuse angles represent far corners and the acute angles near ones or the obtuse angles represent near cor-ners and the acute angles far ones. It is therefore not surprising that the pres-ence or absence of these distortions has nothing to do with depth. The parts of the perspective projection of a rectangle that form obtuse angles are always the most contracted and the parts that form

acute angles are always the most ex-panded. The fact that the obtuse angles have a much larger effect in the Müller-Lyer illusion suggests that constancy scaling tends to equalize lengths by expanding the most contracted parts (bounded by obtuse angles) to match the rest of the projection rather than to diminish the more expanded parts (bounded by acute angles) to match the rest of the projection.

If contraction and expansion illusions serve to compensate for properties of the projection that are not properties of the scene that was projected, then the greater the distortions caused by per-spective projection are, the greater is the illusion needed to compensate for the distortion. That is the case with the Mül-ler-Lyer illusion, which gets stronger as the angles deviate more from right an-gles and as the arrowheads become larg-er. (There is a limit I cannot account for, however, on the effect the size of the arrowheads has on the magnitude of the illusion.)

I want to turn now to the Poggendorff illusion and discuss what it means in terms of perspective. The oblique lines of the Poggendorff figure do not seem to be significantly misaligned when they are viewed alone. Why does insertion of the vertical parallel lines disrupt the ap-parent alignment of the oblique lines to such a great degree? Although collinear lines in the three-dimensional world al-ways project as collinear lines on the retina, noncollinear lines in the three-di-mensional world can also project as col-linear lines. I contend that the parallel lines of the Poggendorff figure, particu-larly the components forming obtuse angles, provide a context suggesting that the oblique lines do not represent collin-ear lines in three-dimensional space. As a result the oblique lines do not appear to be collinear. This is shown in the bot-tom illustration on the opposite page.

From the point of view of perspective, oblique lines represent receding hori-zontal lines. When two oblique lines are lined up, as they are in the Poggendorff illusion, the conventions of perspective dictate that the space between them on the picture plane could represent one of two possible arrangements. The points *B* and *C* in the illustration could repre-sent an interruption in a continuous re-ceding horizontal dimension, in which case the line *ABCD* would lie on a single horizontal plane in three-dimensional space. The other possibility is that *B* and *C* represent points that are separat-ed both horizontally and vertically, in which case *AB* and *BC* would lie on different horizontal planes and would therefore be noncollinear in three-di-mensional space.

Visual processing favors the noncol-linear arrangement when details placed within the gap *BC* are consistent with equidistance rather than with a depth difference for *B* and *C*. The parallel lines of the Poggendorff figure are particularly effective in this regard because they place *B* and *C* on a plane seen head on. What actually seems to happen is that the context changes the arrangement from one in which *AB*, *BC* and *CD* are each seen as having less slope than they do on the picture plane, because they all represent horizontal lines, to one in which the apparent slopes of *AB* and *CD* remain the same, because they continue to represent horizontal lines, whereas the apparent slope of *BC* increases, because it no longer represents a horizontal line. The result is a disruption of perceived collinearity. This explanation is supported experimentally by the work of Ross H. Day and R. G. Dickinson of Monash University in Australia, who asked experimental subjects to estimate the slopes of *AB*, *BC* and *CD* in the Poggendorff figure.

A consequence of my explanation of the Poggendorff figure is that the illusion should be greatly reduced if the length of the parallel lines is changed so that they outline not a plane seen head on but an appropriately receding plane, in which case *AB*, *BC* and *CD* are collinear in three-dimensional space. This change can be achieved by making the ends of the parallel lines and the oblique lines converge on a single vanishing point. When the vanishing point is clearly defined, the magnitude of the illusion is reduced by half. This provides strong evidence that the context relevant to the three-dimensional layout represented by two-dimensional lines strongly influences the perceived collinearity.

The evaluation of a functional theory based on perspective decoding is hampered by the fact that so little is known about perceptual responses to perspective, in spite of the fact that much of Western art has been based on perspective for 500 years. It is unlikely, however, that all illusions are the result of perspective decoding. For example, no obvious constancy function is served by illusions of orientation assimilation, such as the Lipps figure. Yet my functional theory, unlike the other theories, can handle in a general way the maintenance of illusory responses under normal three-dimensional viewing conditions, where the responses are reinforced because they promote accurate perception, and the diminution of illusory responses under two-dimensional viewing conditions, where the responses are inhibited because they serve no function.

W ork remains to be done on how the diminution is achieved and on what role eye movements play in the process. Stanley Coren of the University of British Columbia and Joan S. Girgus of Princeton University have proposed

that illusions that strongly diminish in the course of repeated exposure have a considerable judgmental or learned component, whereas illusions that only weakly diminish, for example assimilation illusions such as the Delboeuf one,

are chiefly built in. Although constancy responses are traditionally regarded as being based on learned algorithms, there is no reason some of the responses could not be built-in ones that evolved because they promoted constancy. In principle

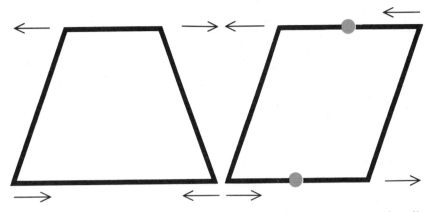

QUADRANGLES ON THE RETINA are usually the projections of rectangles in three-dimensional space. A perceptual mechanism that lengthens horizontal lines bounded by obtuse angles and shortens horizontal lines bounded by acute angles would compensate for the difference in size caused by perspective projection. The arrows indicate the direction of the perceptual expansion or contraction. The colored dots mark the midpoints of the horizontal lines of the quadrangle at the right. The midpoints appear to be too close to perceptually shortened ends.

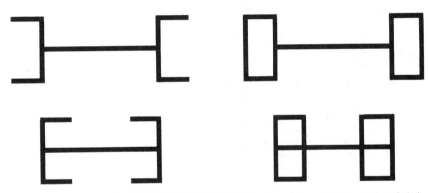

RECTANGULAR MÜLLER-LYER FIGURES (*left*) also create an illusion, although it is much weaker than the one created by the normal Müller-Lyer figures that are shown in the illustration on page 103. The illusion gets quite strong when the appendages are closed up to form rectangles (*right*). No theory of geometrical illusions can account for this phenomenon.

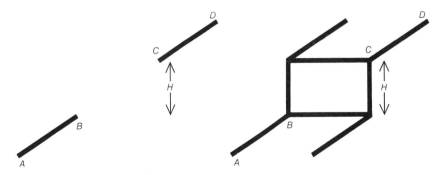

COLLINEAR LINES ON THE RETINA need not necessarily represent collinear lines in three-dimensional space. The points *B* and *C* at the left could represent an interruption in a continuous receding horizontal dimension, in which case the line *ABCD* would lie on a single horizontal plane in three-dimensional space. The other possibility (*right*) is that *B* and *C* represent points that are separated both horizontally and vertically, in which case *AB* and *CD* would lie on different horizontal planes and would therefore be noncollinear in three-dimensional space. The presence of parallel vertical lines in the Poggendorff figure favors the arrangement at the right, and so the visual system interprets the lines *AB* and *CD* as having different heights.

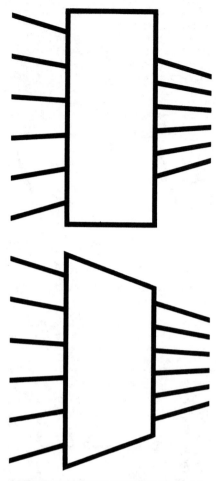

ORIENTATION OF THE PLANE strongly alters an illusion for a set of collinear oblique lines with a common vanishing point. The top lines, which interrupt a plane seen head on, appear to deviate more from being collinear than the bottom lines, which interrupt a receding plane that has the same vanishing point as the lines. This provides evidence that the context relevant to the three-dimensional layout represented by lines in two dimensions strongly influences the perceived collinearity.

theories emphasizing function are not incompatible with theories emphasizing mechanism.

Functional theories based on perspective are supported to some degree by responses to geometrical illusions among peoples who do not live in a world dominated by rectangular rooms, buildings and cities. For such people the illusions tend to be not as strong as they are for people in our own kind of culture. Their response to the upside-down-T illusion, on the other hand, which seems to depend not on the exposure to a rectangular environment but on the foreshortening of distant terrain, is not reduced. Striking as such results are, they should not be allowed to carry much theoretical weight until it is clear the people involved in the experiments have had the same understanding of what it is they are being asked to do as subjects in our own kind of culture. If such results hold up, however, they could significantly bolster the functional theories.

Perhaps the most serious challenge to functional theories, and for that matter to all theories of illusion relying on processes in the visual system, could come from investigations into the sense of touch. Experiments have revealed touch illusions that are analogous to optical ones when subjects ran their fingers over raised versions of well-known illusory figures. At this stage, however, the work is too tentative to establish any identity between misperceptions of touch and misperceptions of vision.

10

The Interpretation of Visual Illusions

by Donald D. Hoffman
December 1983

The visual system apparently organizes ambiguous retinal images according to rules of inference that exploit certain regularities in the external world

Vision is a process of inference. What you see when you look around depends not only on what is there to be seen but also on how your visual system organizes and interprets the images that fall on your retinas. An intriguing demonstration of this aspect of perception is presented by the apparent surface that is formed by rotating a cosine wave around a vertical axis viewed obliquely [*see illustration on this page*]. When you first look at the figure, it appears to be organized into a set of raised concentric rings, with the boundaries between the rings delineated approximately by the colored circular contours. If you turn the page upside down, however, the organization changes: now each colored contour, instead of lying in a trough between two rings, appears to trace the crest of a ring. (Try it.) Evidently the visual system does more than passively transmit signals to the brain. It actively takes part in organizing and interpreting them.

This finding raises three questions. First, why does the visual system need to organize and interpret the images formed on the retinas? Second, how does it remain true to the real world in the process? Third, what rules of inference does it follow? The answers to these questions call for a closer examination of such figures.

One reason the visual system organizes and interprets retinal images is simply that many possible configurations in the real world are consistent with any given retinal image. In other words, retinal images need organization and interpretation because they are fundamentally ambiguous. Their ambiguity is due in part to the fact that the world is three-dimensional and each retina is essentially two-dimensional. To describe the world in its full three-dimensional glory necessarily involves some rather sophisticated inferences by the visual system, inferences that for the most part proceed without any conscious awareness. For example, the cosine surface at the right, like your retinal image of it, is two-dimensional. Yet it appears, quite compellingly, as three-dimensional. The appearance of depth is entirely inferred, or, to put it another way, hallucinated. This conclusion should be cause for some concern. If, as I suggest, such hallucinations are not an exception but the rule, and if they are in fact a necessary concomitant of visual perception, how can one justify one's faith in perception? How is it still possible that in general seeing is believing?

What is needed for an understanding of vision, therefore, is an explanation of why such visual inferences usually bear a nonarbitrary relation to the real world. A promising line of investigation begins with the observation that the visible world, far from being completely chaotic, obeys certain laws and exhibits numerous regularities. If the visual system is adapted to exploit these laws and regularities in its organization and interpretation of retinal images, and if it is constrained somehow to prefer the interpretation that is most credible, given both the image and a knowledge of these laws and regularities, then it might be possible to understand how it is that one's visual hallucinations bear a nonarbitrary and even useful relation to the external world.

A particularly clear example of this approach is the research into visual mo-

AMBIGUOUS SURFACE is made by rotating a cosine wave about a vertical axis. The surface initially appears to be organized into raised concentric rings, with the colored circular contours lying in the troughs between the rings. When the page is turned upside down, however, the organization appears to change: each colored contour is now seen to trace the crest of a ring.

tion perception done by Shimon Ullman of the Massachusetts Institute of Technology. Ullman has explored the remarkable ability of the human visual system to perceive the correct three-dimensional structure and motion of an object solely from its moving two-dimensional projection, an ability Hans Wallach and Donald N. O'Connell of Swarthmore College call the kinetic-depth effect. For instance, if a transparent beach ball with tiny light bulbs mounted randomly on its surface is set spinning in a dark room, one immediately perceives the correct spherical layout of the lights [see upper illustration below]. When the spinning stops, so does the perception of the spherical array. How does one see the correct three-dimensional structure when infinitely many three-dimensional structures are consistent with the moving two-dimensional retinal projection? Ullman showed mathematically that if the visual sys-

tem exploits the laws of projection, and if it exploits the fact that the world contains rigid objects, then in principle a unique and correct interpretation can be obtained. In particular he showed that three views of four noncoplanar light bulbs are enough to solve the problem. The key point is that an inference rule, based on a law (the law of projection) and a regularity (namely the fact that the world includes rigid objects), enables the visual system to make a correct interpretation.

At this stage, however, a puzzle arises. The same mathematical precision that shows the rigidity regularity is sufficient in principle to interpret the rotating beach ball also shows the rigidity regularity by itself is insufficient to interpret a similar display. This display was first devised by Gunnar Johansson of the University of Uppsala as an example of what he calls biological motion [see "Visual Motion Perception," by Gun-

nar Johansson; SCIENTIFIC AMERICAN, June, 1975]. Johansson put small light bulbs on the major joints of a person and took motion pictures as the person moved about in a dark room. A single frame of such a film looks like a random collection of white dots on a black background. When the film is set in motion, however, one immediately sees the correct three-dimensional structure of the dots and recognizes that there is an invisible person walking about [see lower illustration below].

When my colleague Bruce E. Flinchbaugh, who is now at Bell Laboratories, and I considered this problem, what puzzled us was that it is possible to see the correct three-dimensional structure even though, according to Ullman's results, one lacks the appropriate information to do so. To infer a correct three-dimensional structure on the basis of the rigidity regularity it is necessary to have three snapshots of at least four nonco-

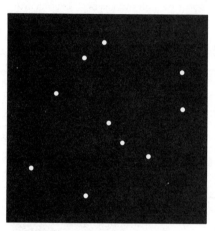 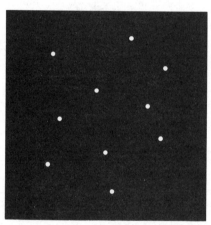 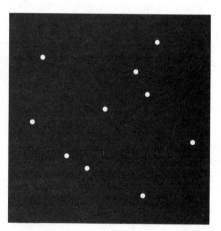

ROTATING SPHERE is seen when the three dot patterns represented here are shown in rapid succession. The visual system seems to be adopting the most rigid three-dimensional interpretation for the moving dots that is consistent with the two-dimensional projections.

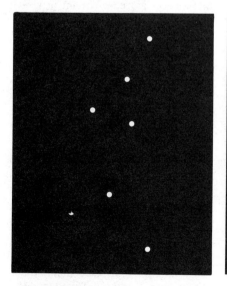 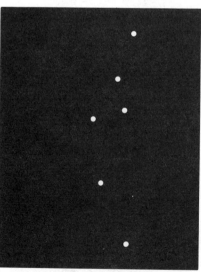 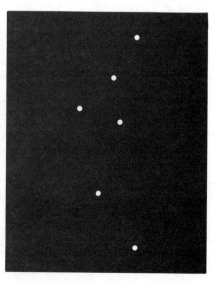

WALKING PERSON is seen when these dot patterns are shown in rapid succession. In this case the visual system seems to adopt the most rigid and planar three-dimensional interpretation that is consistent with the two-dimensional motions of the dots. The display is based on an experiment conducted by Gunnar Johansson of the University of Uppsala in which small light bulbs were put on a person's major joints (shoulder, elbow, wrist, hip, knee and ankle) and a motion picture was made as the person moved about in a dark room.

planar points in a rigid configuration. In biological motion displays, on the other hand, at best only pairs of points are rigidly connected, such as the ankle and the knee or the knee and the hip. Rigid quadruplets of points just do not exist.

The rigidity regularity, then, is insufficient by itself, leading us to ask: What further regularity might the visual system be exploiting? After several false starts it occurred to us there is an anatomical regularity that might do the trick. Each weight-bearing limb of most animals is constrained, because of the construction of its joints, to swing in a single plane in a normal gait. We call this the planarity regularity.

In fact, the planarity regularity is sufficient to correctly interpret biological-motion displays of gait. The correct three-dimensional structure can be inferred either from three snapshots of two points swinging rigidly in a plane or from two snapshots of three points (such as an ankle, a knee and a hip) forming rigid pairs and swinging in one plane. These results comport nicely with Johansson's observation that only two or three frames of his films need be seen before subjects correctly perceive the biological motion. In addition it turns out not only that all three-dimensional motions governed by the planarity regularity can be given a correct interpretation but also that whenever an interpretation is found for image motion based on the planarity regularity or the rigidity regularity the interpretation is correct.

In short, the probability that the interpretation is wrong is zero, assuming infinite resolution in the image, or slightly greater than zero given less than perfect resolution. Hence nonrigid structures cannot masquerade as rigid ones, and nonplanar motions cannot be misconstrued as planar ones. Once again laws and regularities prove to be central in explaining how the visual system achieves a unique and correct interpretation of a retinal image.

Let us now return to the cosine surface. Its main interest is that it reveals the visual system organizing shapes into parts, an organization that is quite useful for the task of recognizing an object from its shape. The cosine surface also reveals that turning a shape upside down can alter this organization. Is the visual system, then, capricious in its organization? That is unlikely. If it is not governed by whim, however, it must be governed by rules for defining parts. And if the rules are not to be arbitrary, they must be grounded in some law or regularity in the external world.

This line of reasoning led Whitman A. Richards of M.I.T. and me to seek a law or regularity that could motivate a set of rules for partitioning surfaces. The regularity we found to be relevant is the following transversality regularity:

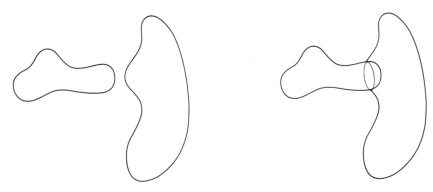

TRANSVERSALITY, a kind of regularity commonly observed in the external world, underlies a unified account of several visual illusions. According to the rule of transversality (as defined by Whitman A. Richards and the author), when any two surfaces penetrate each other at random, they always meet at a concave discontinuity, indicated here by the colored contour.

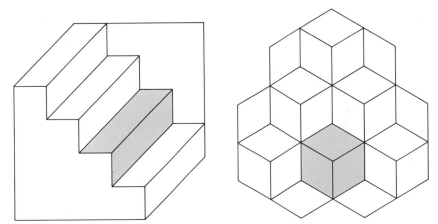

PARTITIONING RULE based on the transversality regularity is demonstrated with the aid of these two figures that reverse when they are looked at steadily. In both cases the apparent boundaries of the different parts of the perceived shape change when the "figure" becomes the "ground" and vice versa. For example, in the case of the reversing-stairway illusion (*left*), first published by H. Schröder in 1858, the two colored panels, which in one view appear to be parts of one step, suddenly seem to be parts of two adjacent steps when the stairway reverses. Similarly, in the stacked-cube illusion (*right*) the three diamond-shaped colored panels can be seen either as the faces of one cube or, when the figure reverses, as the faces of three different cubes.

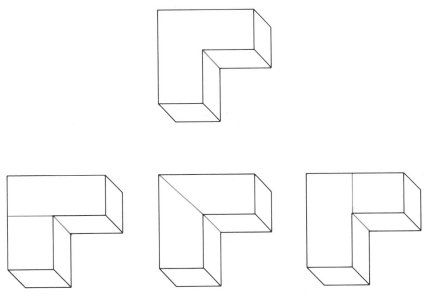

ELBOW-SHAPED BLOCKS show that the rule partitioning shapes at concave discontinuities is appropriately conservative. The rule does not give a closed contour on the top block because three different perceived partitions seem possible, as illustrated by the bottom three blocks.

When two arbitrarily shaped surfaces are made to penetrate each other at random, they always meet at a contour of concave discontinuity of their tangent planes [*see top illustration on page 97*]. Although the transversality regularity may sound esoteric, it is actually a familiar part of everyday experience. A straw in a soft drink, for instance, forms a circular concave discontinuity where it meets the surface of the drink. A candle in a birthday cake, the tines of a fork in a piece of steak, a cigarette in a mouth—all are examples of this ubiquitous regularity.

On the basis of the transversality regularity one can propose a first rule for partitioning a surface: Divide a surface into parts along all contours of concave discontinuity. This rule cannot help with the cosine surface because it is entirely smooth. The rule must first be generalized somewhat, as will be done below. In its nongeneralized form, however, it can elucidate several well-known perceptual demonstrations.

For example, the rule makes the obvious prediction that the parts of the staircase shown in the middle illustration on page 97 are its steps, each step lying between two successive lines of concave discontinuity in the staircase. The rule also makes a less obvious prediction. If the staircase undergoes a perceptual reversal, such that the "figure" side becomes "ground" and vice versa, then the step boundaries must change. This conclusion follows because only concave discontinuities define the step boundaries, and what looks like a concavity from one side of a surface must look like a convexity from the other. Thus when the staircase reverses, convex and concave discontinuities must reverse roles, leading to new step boundaries. You can test this prediction yourself by looking at the step that has color on each of its two faces. When the staircase appears to reverse, note that the colored panels are no longer on a single step but rather on adjacent steps.

This prediction can be confirmed with a more complicated demonstration such as the stacked-cubes test seen in the same illustration. The three colored faces, which at first appear to be on one cube, are seen to be on three cubes when the figure reverses.

A further prediction follows from this simple partitioning rule. If the rule does not define a unique partition of some surface, then the appropriate way to divide the surface into parts should be perceptually ambiguous (unless there are additional rules that can eliminate the ambiguity). A clear confirmation of this prediction can be seen with reference to the elbow-shaped block in the bottom illustration on page 97. The only concave discontinuity is the vertical line in the crook of the elbow. As a

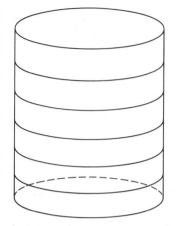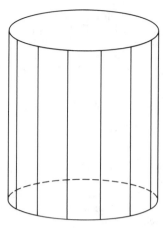

LINES OF CURVATURE are easily pictured on an idealized cylindrical drinking glass. The lines of greatest curvature (*left*) are circles; the lines of least curvature (*right*) are straight lines.

consequence the rule does not define a unique partition of the block. Perceptually there are three plausible ways to cut the block into parts. All three ways rely on the contour defined by the partitioning rule, but they complete it along different paths.

Even this simple partitioning rule leads to interesting insights into the perception of shape. To explore the cosine surface and other smooth surfaces, however, the rule must be generalized. This requires a brief digression into the differential geometry of surfaces in order to understand three important concepts: surface normal, principal curvature and line of curvature. Fortunately, although these concepts are quite technical, they can readily be given an intuitive characterization.

The surface normal at a point on a surface can be thought of as a needle of unit length sticking straight out of the surface at that point, much like the spines on a sea urchin. All the surface normals at all points on a surface are collectively called a field of surface normals. Usually there are two possible fields of surface normals on a surface; they can be either outward-pointing or inward-pointing. For example, a sphere can have the surface normals all pointing radially out like spines or all pointing in toward its center. Let us adopt the convention that the field of surface normals is always chosen to point into the figure. Thus a baseball has inward normals whereas a bubble under water has outward normals. Reversing the choice of figure and ground on a surface im-

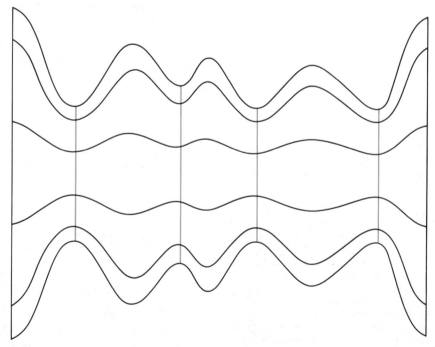

PART BOUNDARIES, as defined by the generalized, smooth-surface partitioning rule, are represented by the colored contours on this arbitrarily shaped surface. The black lines are the lines of greatest curvature whose minimums give rise to the colored partitioning contours.

plies a·concomitant change in the surface normals. A reversal of the field of surface normals induces a change in sign of each of the principal curvatures at every point on the surface.

It is often important to know not only the surface normal at a point but also how the surface is curving at the point. The 18th-century Swiss mathematician Leonhard Euler discovered that at any point on any surface there is always a direction in which the surface curves the least and a second direction, always at right angles to the first, in which the surface curves the most. (In the case of a plane or a sphere the surface curvature is identical in all directions at every point.) These two directions are called principal directions, and the corresponding surface curvatures are called principal curvatures. By starting at some point and always moving in the direction of the greatest principal curvature one traces out a line of greatest curvature. By moving instead in the direction of the least principal curvature one traces out a line of least curvature. On a drinking glass the family of lines of greatest curvature is a set of circles around the glass. The lines of least curvature are straight lines running the

length of the glass [*see top illustration on preceding page*].

With these concepts in mind the transversality regularity extends easily to smooth surfaces. Suppose wherever a surface has a concave discontinuity one smoothes the discontinuity somewhat, perhaps by stretching a taut skin over it. Then a concave discontinuity becomes, roughly speaking, a contour where the surface has locally the greatest negative curvature. More precisely, the generalized version of transversality suggests the following generalized partitioning rule for surfaces: Divide a surface into parts at negative minimums of each principal curvature along its associated family of lines of curvature [*see bottom illustration on preceding page*].

This rule partitions the cosine surface along the colored circular contours. It also explains why the parts are different when the page is turned upside down: the visual system then reverses its assignment of figure and ground on the surface (perhaps owing to a preference for an interpretation that places the object below the observer's viewpoint rather than above it). When figure and ground reverse, so does the field of surface normals, in accordance with the convention mentioned above. Simple

calculations show, however, that when the normals reverse, so does the sign of the principal curvatures. As a result minimums of the principal curvatures must become maximums and vice versa. Since minimums of the principal curvatures are used for part boundaries, it follows that these part boundaries must also move. In sum, parts appear to change because the partitioning rule, motivated by the transversality regularity, uses minimums of the principal curvatures, and because these minimums relocate on the surface when figure and ground reverse.

The transversality regularity, in short, provides an underlying unity for explanatory accounts of the perception of parts in both smooth and rough surfaces. It also underlies an explanation of another well-known class of visual illusions: reversing plane curves. A good example of this phenomenon is the reversing figure devised by Fred Attneave of the University of Oregon [*see upper illustration on this page*]. He found that by simply scribbling a line through a circle and separating the two halves one can create two very different-looking contours. Evidently, as Attneave points out, the appearance of the contour depends on which side is taken to be part of the figure, not on any prior familiarity with the contour [see "Multistability in Perception," by Fred Attneave; SCIENTIFIC AMERICAN, December, 1971].

How does the transversality regularity explain this phenomenon? The answer involves three steps: (1) a projection of the transversality regularity from three dimensions onto two dimensions, (2) a brief digression on the differential geometry of plane curves and (3) the formulation of a partitioning rule for plane curves.

The two-dimensional version of the transversality regularity is similar to the three-dimensional version. If two arbitrarily shaped surfaces are made to penetrate each other at random, then in any two-dimensional projection of their composite surface they will always meet in concave cusps. To paraphrase it loosely, concave cusps are always formed in a silhouette at points where one part stops and another begins. This suggests the following partitioning rule for plane curves: Divide a plane curve into parts at concave cusps. This rule cannot apply to Attneave's demonstration because his demonstration relies on a contour that is everywhere smooth. The rule must again be generalized. Nevertheless, in its nongeneralized form it can account for a version of Attneave's demonstration that is not everywhere smooth.

In the lower illustration at the left the same jagged contour can look either like an alternating chain of tall and short mountains or, for the reversed

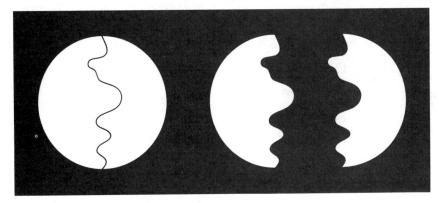

REVERSING PLANE CURVE, constructed by Fred Attneave of the University of Oregon by scribbling a line through a circle and separating the two halves, shows that the apparent shape of the resulting contour depends on which side of the line is perceived as the figure.

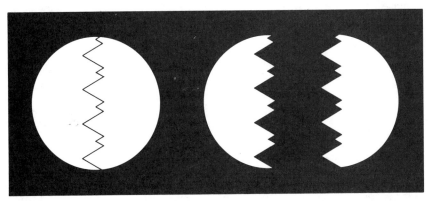

SIMILAR REVERSING FIGURE can be made with a plane curve that is not smooth. One can see the resulting jagged contour either as an alternating chain of tall and short mountains or, in the reversed figure-ground assignment, as a chain of tall mountains with twin peaks.

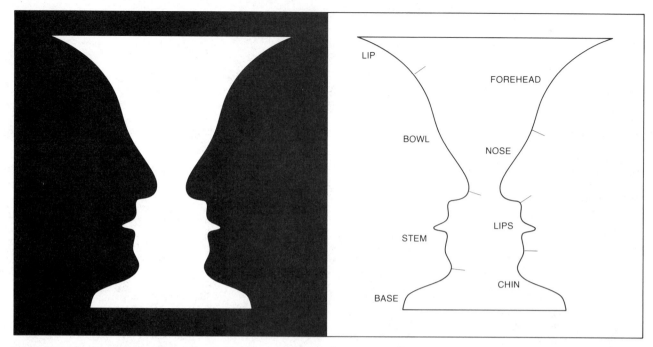

FACE-GOBLET ILLUSION, devised by Edgar Rubin in about 1915, can be seen either as a pair of facial profiles or as a goblet (*left*). If a face is taken to be the figure, partitioning the figure by reference to minimums of curvature divides the contour into chunks correspond- **ing to a forehead, a nose, a pair of lips and a chin; if the goblet is taken to be the figure, defining the part boundaries by minimums of curvature divides the contour into a lip, a bowl, a stem and a base (*right*). Principal-normal lines in both cases point into the figure.**

figure-ground assignment, like a chain of tall mountains with twin peaks. The contour is carved into parts differently when figure and ground reverse because the partitioning rule uses only concave cusps for part boundaries. What is a concave cusp if one side of the contour is figure must become a convex cusp when the other side is figure, and vice versa. There is a parallel between this example and the reversible staircase discussed above.

Before generalizing the rule to smooth contours let us briefly review two concepts from the differential geometry of plane curves: principal normal and curvature. The principal normal at a point on a curve can be thought of as a unit-length needle sticking straight out of the curve at that point. All the principal normals at all points on a curve together form a field of principal normals. Usually there are two possible fields of principal normals, one field on each side of the curve. Let us adopt the convention that the field of principal normals is always chosen to point into the figure side of the curve. Reversing the choice of figure and ground on a curve implies a concomitant change in the field of principal normals. What is important to note is that because of the convention forcing the principal normals to point into the figure, concave parts of a smooth curve have negative curvature and convex parts have positive curvature.

It is an easy matter now to generalize the partitioning rule for plane curves. Suppose wherever a curve has a concave

cusp one smoothes the curve a bit. Then a concave cusp becomes a point of negative curvature having, locally, the greatest absolute value of curvature. This observation leads to the following generalized partitioning rule: Divide a plane curve into parts at negative minimums of curvature.

Now it is possible to explain why the two halves of Attneave's circle look so different. When figure and ground reverse, the field of principal normals also reverses in accordance with the convention, and when the principal normals reverse, the curvature at every point on the curve must change sign. In particular, minimums of curvature must become maximums and vice versa. This repositioning of the minimums of curvature leads to a new partitioning of the curve by the partitioning rule. In short, the curve looks different because it is organized into fundamentally different chunks, or units. Note that if one chooses to define part boundaries by inflections, or by both maximums and minimums of curvature, then the chunks would not change when figure and ground reverse.

A clear example of two very different partitions for one curve can be seen in the famous face-goblet illusion devised by Edgar Rubin in about 1915 [*see illustration above*]. If a face is taken to be figure, the minimums of curvature divide the curve into chunks corresponding to a forehead, nose, upper lip, lower lip and chin. If instead the goblet is taken to be figure, the minimums are repo-

sitioned, dividing the curve into new chunks corresponding to a base, a couple of parts of the stem, a bowl and a lip on the bowl. It is probably no accident that the parts defined by minimums are often easily assigned verbal labels.

Demonstrations have been devised that, like the face-goblet illusion, allow more than one interpretation of a single contour but that do not involve a figure-ground reversal. A popular example is the rabbit-duck illusion [*see top illustration on next page*]. Because such illusions do not involve a figure-ground reversal, and because as a result the minimums of curvature never change position, the partitioning rule must predict that the part boundaries are identical for both interpretations of each of the contours. This prediction is easily confirmed. What is an ear on the rabbit, say, becomes part of a bill on the duck.

If the minimums rule for partitioning curves is really obeyed by the human visual system, one would expect it to predict some judgments of shape similarity. One case in which its prediction is counterintuitive can be seen in the bottom illustration on the next page. Look briefly at the single half-moon on the left side of the illustration. Then look quickly at the two half-moons at the right and decide which one seems more like the first one. In an experiment done on several similar figures, Aaron F. Bobick of M.I.T. and I found that almost all subjects chose the half-moon at the lower right as the more similar one. Yet if you look again, you will find that the bounding contour for the half-moon at

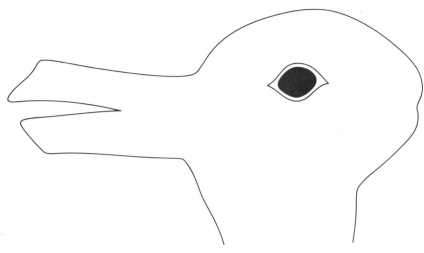

REVERSING-ANIMAL ILLUSION does not involve a reversal of figure and ground. Accordingly the part boundaries defined by the minimums of curvature do not change position when the interpretation changes. The rabbit's ears turn into the duck's bill without moving.

the upper right is identical with that of the left half-moon, only it is figure-ground reversed. The bounding contour of the lower half-moon has been mirror reversed, and two parts defined by minimums of curvature have been swapped. Why does the lower one still look more similar? The minimums rule gives a simple answer. The lower contour, which is not figure-ground reversed from the original contour, has the same part boundaries. The upper contour, which is figure-ground reversed from the original, has different part boundaries.

In summary, vision is an active process whose function is to infer useful descriptions of the world from changing patterns of light falling on the retinas. These descriptions are reliable only to the extent that the inferential processes building them exploit regularities in the visual world, such as rigidity, planarity and transversality. The discovery of relevant regularities and the mathematical investigation of their power in guiding visual inferences are promising directions for the investigator seeking an understanding of human vision.

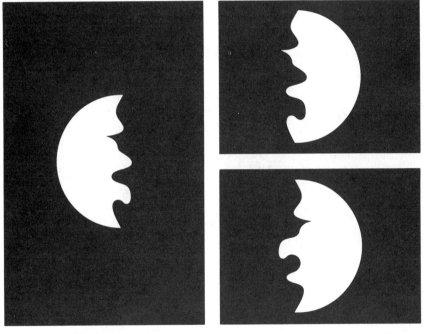

HALF-MOON TEST demonstrates that judgments of the similarity of shapes can be correctly predicted by the minimums-of-curvature partitioning rule. At first glance the half-moon at the lower right seems to resemble the single half-moon at the left more than the one at the upper right does. Closer inspection, however, reveals that the bounding contour of the upper-right half-moon is identical with that of the half-moon at the left, whereas the bounding contour of the lower-right half-moon has been mirror reversed and has also had two parts interchanged.

11 Turning Something Over in the Mind

by Lynn A. Cooper and Roger N. Shepard
December 1984

*The imagined rotation of an object mirrors a physical rotation.
The mental process can be investigated objectively, yielding
quantitative information about one form of spatial thinking*

What is thinking? Introspection supplies preliminary answers. Some thought is verbal: a kind of silent talking to oneself. Other mental processes seem to be visual: images are called to mind and wordlessly manipulated. Evident though they are, the mechanisms of thought long eluded experimental analysis and quantification. How can these seemingly inaccessible, subjective processes be measured and investigated scientifically?

We have begun to provide an answer to this question by devising experiments to probe the nature of one mode of thinking: imagined spatial operations. Our results confirm empirically what is subjectively apparent: that the mind can model physical processes, subjecting them to the geometric constraints that hold in the external world. Evidence of such mental operations abounds in everyday life. Consider this question: How do you take a card table through a narrow doorway without folding up its legs? Most people report that they must

envision the process of turning the table on its side, putting two of the legs into the opening, then turning and moving the table so that the legs, the top and the other pair of legs pass through the door.

This kind of spatial imagination may not be peculiar to human beings. One of us witnessed a German shepherd retrieving a long stick that had been thrown over a fence from which one vertical board was missing. The dog bounded through the gap, seized the stick in its mouth and plunged headlong back toward the narrow opening. Just as catastrophe seemed imminent the dog stopped short, paused and rotated its head 90 degrees. With the stick held vertically it passed through the fence without mishap. The operation that took place in the mind of the dog in the moment before it turned its head presumably was not verbal. Might it not have been a preparatory mental rotation of the stick? (And was it not by spatial visualization rather than verbal deduction that you, the reader, understood how ca-

tastrophe threatened and was averted?)

The ability to represent objects or arrangements of objects and their transformations in space clearly is valuable in managing the concrete realities of everyday life, making it possible to plan actions and to anticipate outcomes. It may also play an important role in abstract thought. Many scientists have testified that their greatest achievements grew from imagined spatial relations and transformations. Two well-known cases are Friedrich Kekulé's image of the structure of the benzene molecule and James Watt's visualization of the mechanism of the condensing steam engine. Albert Einstein even remarked that he arrived at the theory of relativity by "visualizing ... effects, consequences and possibilities" through "more or less clear images which can be 'voluntarily' reproduced and combined."

Yet subjective and qualitative assessments, even those made by scientists, cannot substitute for an objective and quantitative understanding. As the distinguished physiological psychologist K. S. Lashley put it in 1923, "introspection may make the preliminary survey, but it must be followed by the chain and transit of objective measurement." Such systematic inquiry into spatial imagination has been slow in arriving.

For the first half of the 20th century theoretical barriers stood in the way. During this time American behaviorists from J. B. Watson to B. F. Skinner tried to sever psychology from its introspective origins in philosophy and establish it on its own empirical foundations. They insisted that all theoretical terms correspond to objectively specifiable stimuli and responses and banished such references to subjective phenomena as the terms consciousness, mind, thinking and imagining. Laboratory studies focused on physically recordable events such as bar pressing by rats and lever pecking by pigeons rather than on the hidden workings of the mind.

During the second half of the century new developments began to erode the barriers the behaviorists had erect-

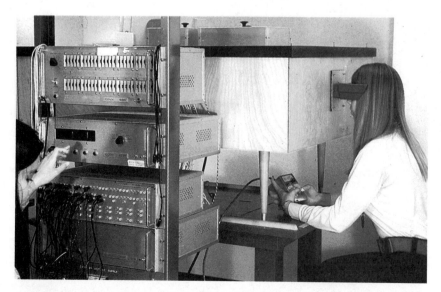

TACHISTOSCOPE enables an investigator to time a subject's responses to visual stimuli. When the investigator closes a switch, a display is illuminated, revealing the images, and a timer begins to run. The subject's reaction, registered in the illustrated case through hand-held controls, stops the clock to yield a precise record of the interval between stimulus and response.

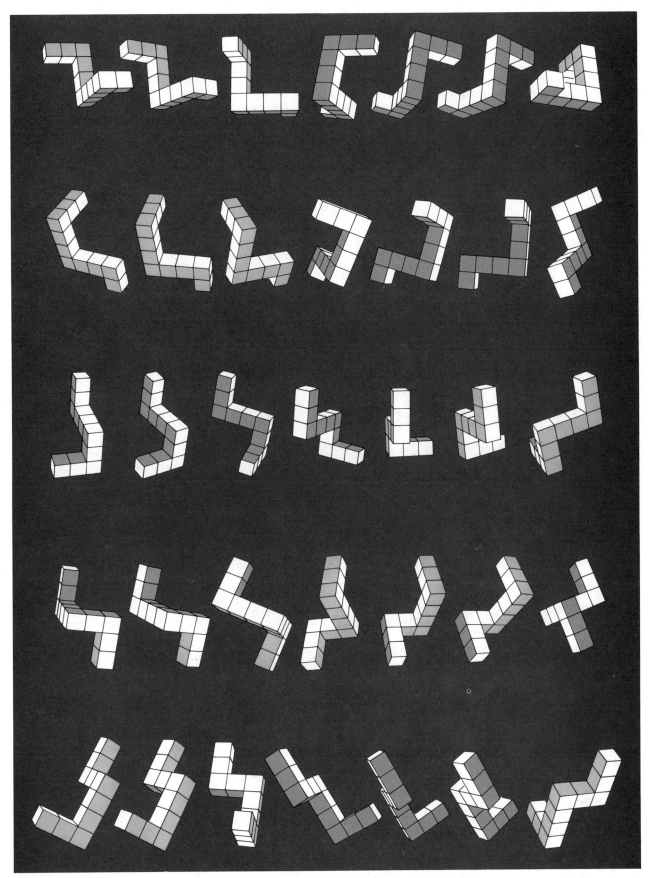

THREE-DIMENSIONAL SHAPES rotated in space are depicted in computer-generated perspective drawings. When the subjects were shown pairs of line drawings portraying the same shape in different orientations, the time they took to recognize that the shapes were identical was proportional to the angular difference in the orientations shown. The linear increase in comparison time with difference in orientation suggested that subjects had to imagine one shape rotated into the orientation of the other in order to check for a match.

ed against the study of the structures and processes of thought. The linguist Noam Chomsky made a forceful argument that language behavior is guided by innate schematisms that had gone completely unrecognized by the behaviorists. And experimental psychologists produced increasingly compelling demonstrations that mental processes could be inferred and even quantified from patterns in objectively recorded data.

Our own experiments were designed to probe the kind of mental process the behaviorists ignored in a way that meets the behaviorists' demand for ob-

jective and quantitative data. The first of our inquiries into the process of spatial imagination, undertaken in 1971 by one of us (Shepard) with Jacqueline Metzler, a graduate student, met both criteria. Each experimental trial was objective in the sense that the subject's response to a stimulus was either objectively correct or incorrect, and quantitative in the sense that the variable of interest was the time it took the subject to respond correctly.

The subjects of the experiment compared computer-generated perspective line drawings presented in pairs. Each drawing portrayed a three-dimensional

object composed of 10 cubical blocks joined face to face to form an armlike structure exhibiting three right-angled bends [*see illustration on page 103*]. Certain of the pairs showed identical structures, usually presented in different spatial orientations; others, randomly mixed with the first type in the series of trials, showed structures that differed in both shape and orientation. These pairs portrayed enantiomorphic structures, which differ by a reflection in space, much as a left hand differs from a right.

In each trial the subject looked into a tachistoscope, a darkened box in which visual stimuli placed at the back could be displayed at precisely controlled times. The experimenter inserted a pair of drawings and closed a switch to illuminate them, simultaneously starting a clock. The subject then compared the drawings as quickly as possible and responded by pulling one of two levers: a right-hand lever for pairs that showed the same shape and a left-hand lever for pairs that showed different shapes. Either response stopped the clock, thus recording the time taken for comparison.

Because the pairs of drawings represented objects that either were identical or differed by a reflection in space, subjects could not base their comparison on superficial features of the stimuli. The numbers of blocks between successive bends, for instance, were identical in both drawings whether the structures were identical or enantiomorphic. A short-cut search for obvious differences was ruled out. Subjects reported they could compare the shapes only by imagining one of the two objects rotated into the same orientation as the other and then checking for a match. Typically they said they imagined the object on the left turned until its top arm paralleled the corresponding arm of the right-hand object; they then mentally checked to see whether the extension at the other end of the object projected in the same direction as the analogous section of the companion structure.

The reaction times, measured from the moment the drawings were displayed until each subject responded by pulling a lever, provide objective evidence in support of the subjective accounts. The times increased as a linear function of the angular difference between the orientations portrayed. When like objects were displayed in the same orientation, subjects took about a second to detect identity; with increasing angular difference the response times rose steadily, up to an average of 4.4 seconds for the maximum possible angular difference of 180 degrees. Each of the eight young adults who took part showed a linear increase in reaction time, but the slope of the function varied among individuals.

The linear increases suggest that the subjects compared the objects by imag-

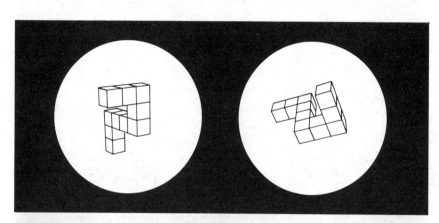

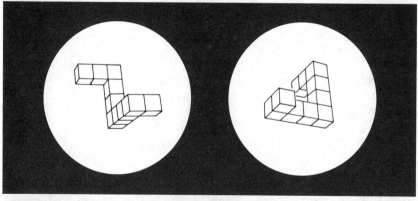

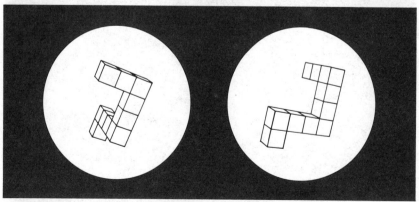

PERSPECTIVE VIEWS displayed in pairs to the subjects of the authors' first experiment differed in three ways. In the first case (*top*) the drawings showed identical objects in positions that differed by a rotation within the plane of the picture. In the second (*middle*) the orientations portrayed differed by a rotation in depth. Subjects determined the identity of the objects in pairs of both types equally quickly, which suggests that in both cases they imagined the objects as three-dimensional solids rotating in space in order to compare them. A third kind of drawing pair used in the trials depicted enantiomorphic, or mirror-image, shapes (*bottom*).

ining one object rotated into the orientation of another at a steady rate that swept out 180 degrees in an average of 3.4 seconds (4.4 minus the second needed to compare two objects in identical orientations), that is, at an average rate of 53 degrees per second. Other methods can be conceived for the discrimination of identical and enantiomorphic objects, but none would take an amount of time proportional to the angular difference. Excluded, for example, is the possibility that subjects analyzed each drawing of a pair separately to reduce its structure to a code of some kind and then compared the coded descriptions. One kind of code might describe the number of blocks and the directions of successive bends, starting at one end of the object: 2R2U2L1 for "two blocks, right bend, two blocks, upward bend, two blocks, left bend, one block," for example. The time needed to generate such a code might depend on the orientation of each object. But because the codes are computed independently, the sum of the times needed to generate codes for two objects need not vary with the angular difference between them.

The results not only point to mental rotation as the basis of this kind of comparison; they also indicate that the subjects' mental images represented the three-dimensional structure of the objects portrayed and not simply the two-dimensional features of the drawings. In half of the same-shape pairs the orientations shown differed by a rotation within the two-dimensional plane of the picture; the two drawings thus were identical except in position in the plane. The other half of the pairs portrayed objects differing by rotations in depth [see illustration on opposite page]. Although the three-dimensional objects depicted by each pair of this second set of drawings were identical, the drawings themselves, as two-dimensional arrangements of lines and angles, often differed considerably: a rotation in depth simultaneously shifts some features of a three-dimensional object into the plane of a drawing while removing other features from the picture plane.

Yet the slope of the reaction-time function was no greater for the pairs corresponding to a rotation in depth than it was for those in which the drawings differed by a picture-plane rotation. The rate of imagined rotation was as fast when the transformation portrayed involved three dimensions as it was when the rotation appeared to take place in two dimensions. The results are consistent with subjects' reports that they interpreted all the drawings, whatever the relative orientations, as solid objects in three-dimensional space. The subjects therefore found all rotations equally easy to imagine.

The progressive and spatial nature of imagined rotations, established in the

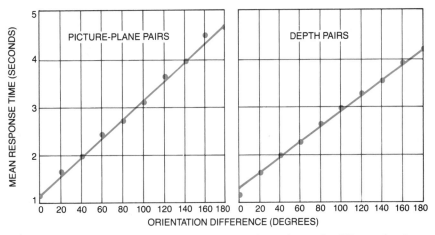

MEAN RESPONSE TIMES increased in direct proportion to the angular difference in orientation of identical objects presented for comparison in pairs of drawings. The linear relation suggested that a process of mental rotation underlies such comparisons. The slope of the function, from which the rate of the imagined rotation can be estimated, was no greater for orientations differing by a rotation in depth than for those differing by a rotation in the picture plane.

first experiment, suggests that the process is analogous to transformations in the physical world. It is tempting to view the imagined rotation as the internal simulation of an external rotation. Such a description, however, would be justified only if we could demonstrate that the internal process passes through intermediate states corresponding to the intermediate orientations of a physical object rotating in the external world.

To gather this additional evidence for the analogue nature of mental rotation one of us (Cooper) did a series of experiments in which subjects responded not to a pair of objects but to a single figure, displayed at intervals and in a variety of orientations. By triggering an imagined rotation with a single stimulus and then presenting the same or a different object in any orientation and after any delay, we could probe the mental transformation as it was taking place.

Before exploring the ongoing process of rotation, however, an initial question required resolution and therefore a brief experimental digression. We had to establish that the single-stimulus technique causes subjects to imagine the same progressive mental rotations as the paired drawings of the first test did. To evaluate the one-stimulus procedure we again asked subjects to discriminate between an object and its mirror image. In this case we used two-dimensional plane figures rather than the three-dimensional solids of the earlier experiment. Consequently all the orientations shown differed by rotations in a plane.

The subjects first learned to differentiate standard from mirror-image versions of each of eight polygons, the orientations of which were kept constant throughout this training [see top illustration on next page]. Once the subjects had learned the eight discriminations the experimental trials began.

In each trial a subject was shown one of the polygons in an orientation that either matched the training position or differed from it by some multiple of 60 degrees. The subject's task was to determine whether the shape was the standard or the reflected version of the polygon; to make the discrimination the subject presumably had to imagine the polygon rotated until it either matched or did not match the mental representation of the standard shape that had been learned during the training. In the case of a match the subject pressed a right-hand button for "standard"; when there was no match, the subject pressed a left-hand button for "reflected."

Like the paired-stimulus procedure, this test yielded a linear increase in reaction time with increasing angular departure—departure, in this case, from a learned position rather than from the orientation of an object displayed simultaneously. Subjects responded to the standard versions of the test polygons a constant 60 milliseconds faster than they did to the reflected versions; it appeared that subjects first compared the transformed test shape with a memory of the standard shape and could react to a match immediately but needed an extra interval to initiate the "reflected" response if the shapes did not correspond.

The slopes of the response-time functions for both standard and reflected test shapes were identical, however. The inferred average rate of mental rotation was 450 degrees per second, considerably higher than the 53 degrees per second estimated in the earlier two-stimulus experiment. Evidently the use of plane images presented one at a time allowed swifter responses by enabling subjects to focus their attention on a single stimulus. In spite of quantitative differences the results of this procedure parallel those of the earlier one.

Having determined that the one-stim-

STANDARD VERSIONS   REFLECTED VERSIONS

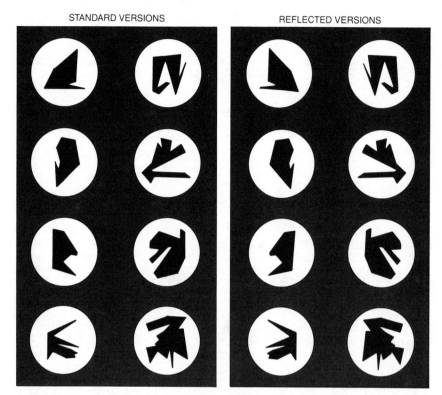

ASSORTMENT OF TWO-DIMENSIONAL TEST SHAPES includes eight different polygons and their mirror-image versions. Prior to a set of experiments in which subjects were shown one of the shapes in an unfamiliar orientation each participant learned to discriminate the "standard" (*left*) from the "reflected" (*right*) version of each shape in a particular orientation. The eight shapes vary in the number of points defining their perimeters, a characteristic that may correspond to psychological complexity. Yet the complexity of a shape had no effect on the speed with which subjects later discriminated its standard form from its reflected form.

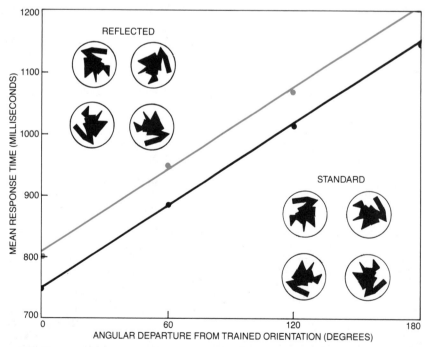

LINEAR RELATION OF RESPONSE TIME TO TEST ORIENTATION was found when subjects viewed a familiar polygon in a new orientation and determined whether it was the standard version (*lower graph*) or the reflected version (*upper graph*) of the shape. To evaluate the test shape subjects apparently had to imagine a rotation of the standard shape until it either matched or did not match the shape displayed. If there was no match, it took subjects a consistent extra increment of time to indicate that the shape before them was the reflected version.

ulus, two-dimensional test requires a mental rotation like that required by the two-stimulus comparison, we could modify the procedure to scrutinize more closely the hypothesis that mental rotation is analogous to rotations in the physical world. The second of the single-stimulus experiments directly tested subjects' statements that they appraised a stimulus by imagining its turning until it matched the learned shape. In effect we reversed the earlier sequence of events: instead of presenting subjects with a stimulus for comparison with a learned shape, thus requiring them to imagine a corrective rotation, we first asked them to imagine the rotation of a learned shape and only then presented a stimulus for comparison.

All the subjects in this experiment had taken part in the earlier one-stimulus experiment and were familiar with the test shapes. In each trial a subject viewed an outline drawing of one of the eight standard polygons that was displayed in the training orientation. The outline was followed by a circle containing a pointer positioned in one of six equally spaced angular increments from zero degrees to 300 degrees of clockwise rotation. The subject then imagined the outlined shape rotated into the orientation indicated by the pointer. In half of the trials the subjects had been instructed to do a clockwise mental rotation; in the other half they had been told to imagine the displayed shape rotated in a counterclockwise direction.

To indicate that the mental operation was complete the subject pressed a button, thus stopping the clock that recorded preparation time. Simultaneously a version of the outlined polygon appeared in the orientation indicated by the arrow and a second clock started. As quickly as possible the subject announced whether the drawing showed the standard or the reflected version of the shape by saying "S" (for "standard") or "R" (for "reflected") into a microphone. A voice-activated relay then stopped the second clock.

Each trial hence yielded two times: the time required to effect the mental rotation and the interval then necessary for the subject to classify a test stimulus. Both sets of results confirmed earlier findings. The time needed for the preparatory mental rotation increased linearly with the angular departure from the training orientation, as earlier results had led us to expect. Moreover, in previous experiments the direction of mental rotation was not specified and the greatest testable rotation was 180 degrees. Here the linear increase in preparation time extended to the maximum clockwise or counterclockwise rotation of 300 degrees, providing further evidence that the mental operation was analogous to a physical rotation. The inferred rate of the preparatory rotations, an average of about 370 degrees per second, was comparable to the 450 degrees per second estimated from the earlier one-stimulus experiment.

The second set of times, which recorded the interval required for subjects to respond to the test stimulus appearing after they signaled readiness, confirmed that the act of mental rotation did in fact prepare them to make the discrimination. On the average they classified each test shape as standard or reflected in less than half a second, regardless of its angular departure from the learned position. If the subjects had needed to do further mental operations after they confronted the test stimulus, response times presumably would have increased with the angular departure of the test stimulus, as they had done in earlier experiments where there was no opportunity for a preparatory mental rotation.

The experiments described so far all document characteristics of completed mental rotations. We found that the time required increases in direct proportion to the angle of rotation, and we confirmed that having imagined a shape rotated into the orientation of a physical stimulus, a subject can determine identity or difference with uniform speed, whatever the degree of rotation. But to characterize the mental process as analogous to physical rotations we still had to show that the mental process passes through stages corresponding to the intermediate angles of a physical rotation. If such a correspondence does exist, the angle at which a displayed shape will elicit the quickest response from an individual who is imagining an ongoing rotation of the shape should change steadily and progressively with time, in step with the mental rotation.

The subjects of a further experiment, designed to test that hypothesis, were all veterans of the two earlier single-stimulus experiments and were familiar with the eight test polygons. On each trial a blank circular field appeared in the tachistoscope and the subject was asked to imagine a specified polygon rotating within the field at the subject's natural rate. After an unpredictable interval that shape or its mirror image appeared; the subject then identified the version as quickly as possible.

Because we already had extensive data on each individual's rate of rotation, we could tailor the trials to the individual subjects. From the earlier experiments we inferred the times and angles at which each subject should be most ready to respond to a test shape. In half of the trials, called the probe-expected trials, the test shape was presented at an angle and time intended to match precisely the ongoing mental rotation. In the other trials the shape was displayed in an orientation that differed by vary-

ing angles from what was calculated to be the orientation imagined at that moment. We termed this second kind of trial probe-unexpected.

If a subject necessarily imagines an object in intermediate orientations in the course of mental rotation, the response to a properly timed and oriented probe should be uniformly fast whatever the angle tested is. The reaction times in the probe-expected trials were consistent with our hypothesis: the response times for trials in which the probe was displayed in an expected orientation were virtually constant at about half a second for every angle.

Another feature of the probe-expected trials is instructive. The orientations

of half of the probes were multiples of 60 degrees—the same orientations that were used in the earlier one-stimulus experiment. The other "expected" probes were displayed at unfamiliar angles, all odd multiples of 30 degrees. If, as we propose, mental rotation does not jump discontinuously from angle to angle but instead progresses steadily through states corresponding to intermediate angles, the response times to properly timed probes in the unfamiliar angles should approximate those for probe angles in which the subjects were well versed. Nearly identical response times at familiar and unfamiliar orientations bore out the hypothesis.

When the probe deviated from the expected orientation, reaction times in-

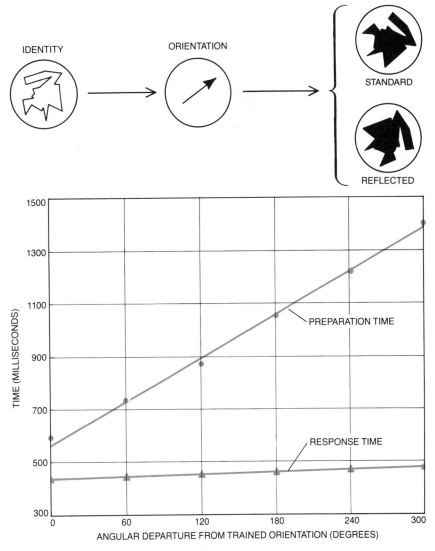

PREPARATORY ROTATION TIMES were measured in the experiment shown schematically at the top; the results are plotted above. Subjects first viewed an outline drawing of one of the eight standard polygons, followed by an arrow. They imagined the shape, now present only in their memory, rotated into the orientation indicated by the arrow. When the mental operation was complete, they signaled by pressing a button, causing a test shape to appear in the designated orientation, and determined as quickly as possible whether the shape was a standard or a reflected version. The time required for the preparatory mental rotation (*upper graph*) increased linearly with the angle; the consistently fast response to the test shape (*lower graph*) confirmed that the process of mental rotation prepared subjects to judge the reoriented shape.

creased linearly with the angle of the discrepancy. Clearly subjects had to imagine a further, correctional rotation when they were presented with a test shape that did not match their current mental representation; the correction took time proportional to the angle of the deviation. The finding provides additional evidence that a correspondence between the imagined and the displayed orientations, and not the subjects' familiarity with the shapes in all orientations, was crucial to the short and constant response times. The correction times indicate that, although the test subjects were practiced, they could not evaluate the displayed shapes without first doing a mental rotation.

Taken together, our results amount to objective evidence of a mental process that models the rotation of objects in the physical world. The two central findings are the linear relation of reaction time to orientation difference when two stimuli are compared for intrinsic shape, and the uniform rapidity of response when a test object is presented in a position calculated to match the steadily changing orientation that is imagined in a mental rotation. We have gathered precise and reproducible data on a seemingly subjective phenomenon of the kind that in the past was considered to lie outside the proper scope of experimental psychology.

Questions still remain about the nature of the mental transformations we have studied. Although we have established that determining the identity of objects displayed in differing orientations can require imagining a rotation through intermediate orientations, we do not contend that the rotation is continuous in the strict mathematical sense, which requires that it sweep through all possible intermediate angles. The neurophysiological basis of the mental images and of their internal manipulation is not known.

Still other questions remain: How much detail from corresponding physical objects do the mental images preserve as they are transformed? Recent experiments suggest that mental representations can preserve much of the structural richness of their material counterparts. In research conducted by Cooper and Peter Podgorny (a former student) subjects were able to discriminate rotated test shapes from standard shapes not only when the probes differed by reflections in space but also when the distinction was a matter of subtle, unpredictable local perturbations [*see bottom illustration at left*].

In spite of some unresolved issues, the close match we have found between mental rotations and their counterparts in the physical world leads inevitably to speculations about the functions and origin of human spatial imagination. It may not be premature to propose that spatial imagination has evolved as a reflection of the physics and geometry of the external world. The rules that govern structures and motions in the physical world may, over evolutionary history, have been incorporated into human perceptual machinery, giving rise to demonstrable correspondences between mental imagery and its physical analogues. We begin to discern here a mental mechanics as precise and elegant as the innate schematism posited by Chomsky as the foundation of language.

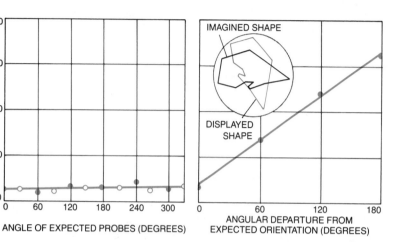

EXPERIMENT PROBING ONGOING MENTAL ROTATIONS yielded the results displayed in the graph. When a subject imagined a shape rotating and the presentation of a test shape was timed so that its orientation matched the momentary orientation of the imagined shape, response times were consistently fast at every angle probed (*left*). The results were not affected by the fact that some of the probes (*open dots*) depicted orientations the subjects had not seen in earlier experiments; instead of skipping between learned positions, objects are imagined as passing through intermediate orientations just as objects rotating in the physical world do. When the investigators deliberately mismatched the probe and the orientation the subject was imagining (*diagram and graph at right*), response times increased with the angular discrepancy. Subjects presumably had to imagine a compensatory rotation to evaluate the test shape.

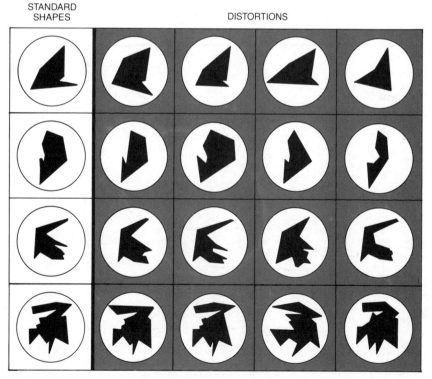

DISTORTIONS OF THE STANDARD SHAPES tested the fidelity with which the features of a physical stimulus are retained when it is rotated mentally. After indicating an orientation into which the subjects were to imagine one of the standard shapes as having rotated, the experimenters presented the reoriented standard shape or one of various distortions of it. Subjects could detect even minor variations from the standard shape, which suggests that in the process of mental rotation much of the structural richness of the original shape is preserved.

Hallucinations

by Ronald K. Siegel
October 1977

*These false perceptions, which can occur in any of the senses,
turn out to be much alike from one person to another.
Apparently they have their roots in excitations of the central
nervous system*

A motorist who drives alone at night in a state of extreme fatigue may well perceive things that are not there: people, animals, vehicles or strange forms. Such a percept is characterized as a hallucination. Although the definition of the word (which comes from the Latin *hallucinari,* meaning to prate, to dream or to wander in mind) is far from precise, one that is widely accepted in psychiatry is: "A false sensory perception in the absence of an actual external stimulus. May be induced by emotional and other factors such as drugs, alcohol and stress. May occur in any of the senses."

By this definition it is likely that everyone has had a hallucination at one time or another. Lonely explorers, isolated hunters in the Arctic and prisoners in dark cells have reported experiencing them. Some people seek out the experience by taking hallucinogenic drugs. Under the right social circumstances the perceptions may be regarded as valid. Joan of Arc became a saint because of her visions, and the flashes of light perceived by the astronauts were taken quite seriously. (They were actually caused by cosmic rays.) On the other hand, negative evaluations are applied to similar perceptions by inmates of correctional institutions. All such reports, however, are necessarily subjective. When one has a hallucination, one does so alone, in the privacy of one's mind.

Do the hallucinations of one person have anything in common with those of another? My colleagues and I in the Neuropsychiatric Institute of the University of California at Los Angeles have attempted to answer the question by means of experiment. We find that hallucinations do have a great deal in common. Moreover, the experiments point to underlying mechanisms in the central nervous system as the source of a universal phenomenology of hallucinations.

One of the earliest classifications of hallucinations was offered in 1853 by Brierre de Boismont of France. He found that hallucinations occurring in states of insanity, delirium tremens, drug intoxication, nervous disorders, nightmares, dreams, ecstasies and fevers were all characterized by excitation and the production of images from memory and the imagination. His countryman Jacques Moreau described hallucinations as being similar to dreams in which imagined visual, auditory and tactile stimuli seem to be real. Foretelling what future neurophysiological research would reveal, he maintained that hallucinations resulted from excitation of the brain. Moreau's technique, which he described in 1845, was to take hashish, which put him in a hallucinatory state while leaving him able to report his experiences. (Moreau also tried to persuade his medical colleagues and friends to take hashish. His colleagues were hesitant because they did not view the taking of hashish as an acceptable form of objective experimentation. The Bohemian artists and writers of 19th-century Paris were more receptive. One of them, the novelist Théophile Gautier, went on to organize the Club des Haschichins, whose members included Balzac, Baudelaire, the younger Dumas and Victor Hugo. Some of the club members' writings testify to the richness of the imagery induced by hashish.)

In Germany and the U.S. early students of hallucinations followed a similar course of self-experimentation and focused mainly on visual hallucinations. Using mescaline, a hallucinogenic alkaloid derived from the peyote cactus *Lophophora williamsii,* Heinrich Klüver began a series of investigations at the University of Chicago in 1926. He reported that mescaline-induced imagery could be observed with the eyes either closed or open and that with the eyes open it was impossible to look at a blank wall without seeing it as being covered with various forms.

Among these forms Klüver found four constant types. One he described with terms such as grating, lattice, fretwork, filigree, honeycomb and chessboard. A second type resembled cobwebs. A third was described with terms such as tunnel, funnel, alley, cone and vessel. The fourth type consisted of spirals. The form constants were further characterized by varied and saturated colors, intense brightness and symmetrical configurations. The visions seemed to be located at reading distance. They varied greatly in apparent size. In general they could not be consciously controlled.

Klüver made the crucial observation that these form constants appear in a wide variety of hallucinatory conditions. He listed a number of the conditions, and other investigators have added to his list, which now includes falling asleep, waking up, insulin hypoglycemia, the delirium of fever, epilepsy, psychotic episodes, advanced syphilis, sensory deprivation, photostimulation, electrical stimulation, crystal gazing, migraine headaches, dizziness and of course a variety of drug intoxications.

Most of the drugs that give rise to such imagery are classifed as hallucinogens. Other drugs and substances can give rise to similar effects, however, and so most psychoactive compounds (to the extent that they cause the mind or the attention to wander) can be regarded as hallucinogens. In this category are alcohol, carbon dioxide, cocaine, cortisol, digitalis, scopolamine and even tobacco with a high concentration of nicotine.

The form constants appear in the first of two stages of drug-induced imagery. The images of the second stage, which are more complex but can incorporate the simple constants, include landscapes, faces and familiar objects and places. The complex images, which are perhaps the most dramatic aspect of the hallucinatory experience, are usually regarded as an activation of images already recorded in the memory.

One would expect the forms and scenes of complex imagery to be almost infinitely diverse. Actually constants appear even at this stage. Indeed, a review of more than 500 hallucinations induced by lysergic acid diethylamide (LSD) revealed that whereas between 62 and 72 percent of the subjects experienced the simple form constants, more than 79 percent reported quite similar complex images. They included religious symbols and images (72 percent) and images of small animals and human beings (49 percent), most of them friendly and many in the nature of cartoons and caricatures.

Most of the investigators and the subjects did not describe the complex imagery in detail. Moreover, before Klüver's classic work little was said about the geometry of even simple hallucinatory images. Klüver attributed this omission to the novelty of the visions, expressing the view that many hallucinating people are so overwhelmed by the color or brightness of the images that they do not articulate the basic forms. It was this inarticulateness that challenged Klüver to describe the simple first stage of hallucinatory imagery. The apparent complexity of the second-stage images challenged us to do the same for them. We believed the study of such phenomena might point to a common visual imagery underlying hallucinations and so might help us understand the origin of these percepts and related ones.

Our first experiments were designed to see if the hallucinatory phenomena I have described appeared when hallucinations were induced in untrained subjects by drugs. Each subject was given either a standard dose of a hallucinogen (usually marihuana or its active principle, tetrahydrocannabinol) or an inactive placebo. (The subject did not know which substance he was receiving.) He was then asked to lie on a bed in a light-proof and soundproof chamber and to report his experiences. We recorded the reports on tape and analyzed them according to the frequency of different

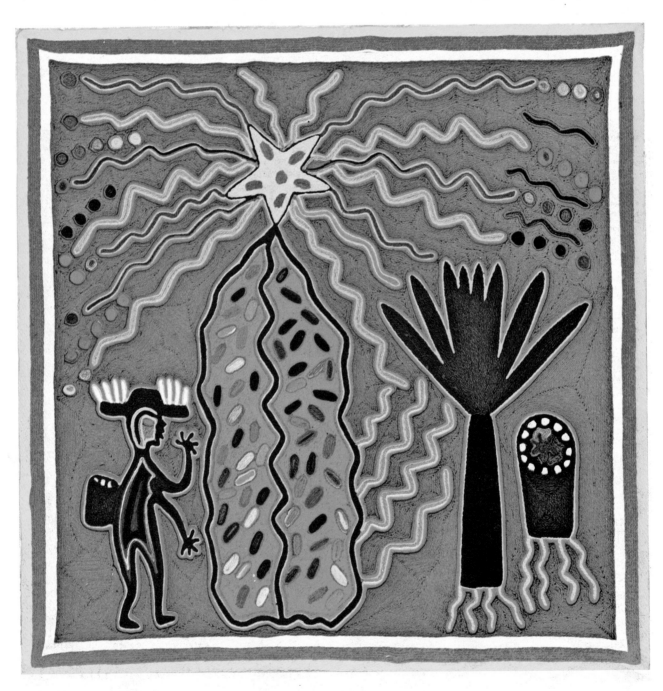

HALLUCINATORY SHAPES AND COLORS are represented in this yarn painting made by a member of the Huichol Indian group in Mexico. The picture was made to show visions of the kind experienced in hallucination brought on by taking peyote. The Indian at the left is carrying a basket of freshly harvested peyote and viewing a vision that is exploding with color and streaks and flashes of light. The peyote cactus is represented at the right. The picture was made by putting beeswax on wood and then pressing yarn into the beeswax.

forms, colors, movements and complex images.

The results showed that normal imagery (that is, imagery not induced by drugs) is characterized by amorphous black-and-white forms (sometimes including lines and curves) that move about randomly in the visual field. Anyone who closes his eyes or goes into a dark room is likely to experience a baseline imagery of this kind. Indeed, one can induce similar imagery, some of it brightly colored and geometric, by gently rubbing one's closed eyelids.

With hallucinogenic drugs, however, the number of images reported by the subjects rose sharply. The consensus was that the imagery resembled what one would see in a motion picture or a slide show. A number of the subjects had difficulty in describing the imagery, but they agreed that there were many geometric forms in it. The imagery was characterized by a bright light in the center of the field of vision that obscured details but allowed images on the periphery to be observed.

The location of this point of light created a tunnel-like perspective. The subjects reported viewing much of their imagery in relation to a tunnel. According to their reports, the images tended to pulsate, moving toward the center of the tunnel or away from the bright light and sometimes moving in both directions.

When the images appeared in color, all colors were reported, although the incidence of reports that the color was red increased as the dosage of the drug increased. Geometric forms frequently combined, duplicated and superimposed. At times the flow of imagery was so rapid that most subjects found it difficult to maintain a running commentary.

The geometric forms were soon replaced by complex imagery. The complex images reported included recognizable scenes, people and objects, many in cartoon or caricature form, with some degree of depth and symmetry. The images were often projected against a background of geometric forms.

In listening to these reports we encountered certain difficulties. The subjects differed widely in their choice of words. Moreover, the reports were riddled with idiosyncratic experiences. We therefore decided to facilitate the ease and accuracy of reporting by training our subjects to use a standard descriptive code.

Efforts along this line had previously been made at Harvard University by the psychologists Ogden R. Lindsley and Timothy Leary. They employed the

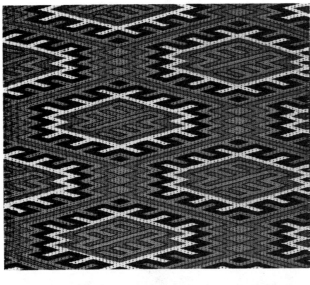

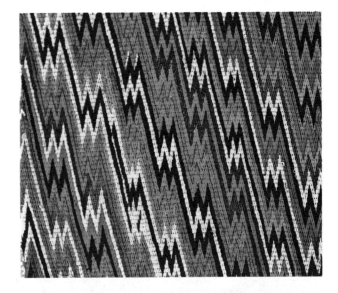

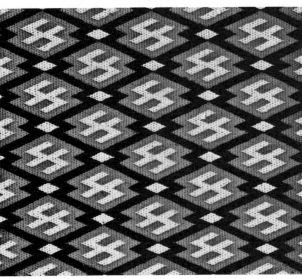

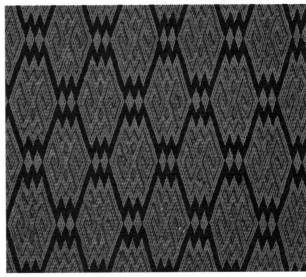

LATTICE FORMS, one of several form constants reported during drug-induced hallucinations, are depicted in four samples of Huichol Indian embroidery. The patterns illustrate designs commonly found in the hallucinatory visions induced by peyote. Some pictures made by schizophrenics exhibit a similar preoccupation with geometric designs, which are often distorted and repeated in symmetrical patterns.

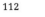

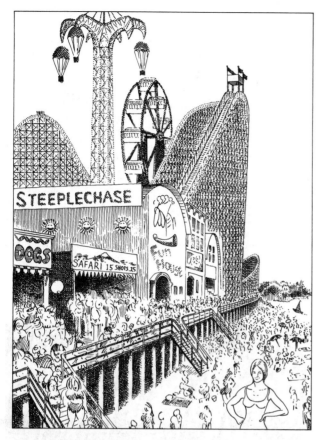

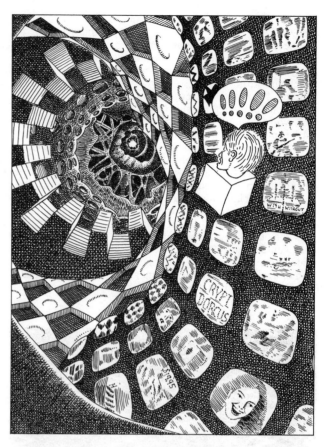

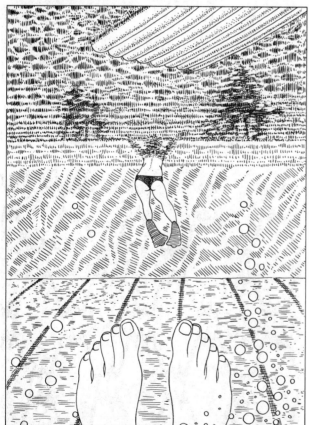

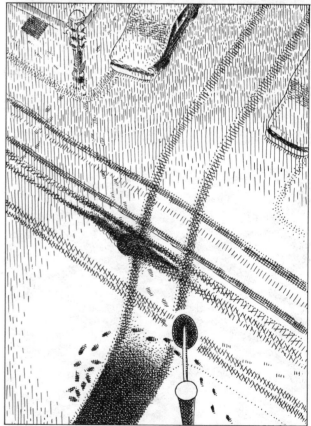

UNUSUAL PERSPECTIVES are reported in hallucinatory images that seem to be drawn from the memory. Characteristic perspectives include a distant scene (with abundant detail) often recognized as an event that was experienced in childhood (*upper left*), a lattice-tunnel pattern with complex memory images at the periphery (*upper right*), a scene viewed as if the subject were under water, looking up toward and through the surface (*lower left*) and an aerial perspective (*lower right*), which may be accompanied by sensations of floating and flying.

operant key press as a reporting device; each key was equated with the occurrence of a subjective state. A hallucinating subject who wanted to report that he "saw" or "heard" something would press a given key for each condition. Lindsley and his colleagues had already demonstrated that the key-pressing technique provided a continuous and objective method for the study of gross behavior in altered states of consciousness.

Nevertheless, a method for obtaining detailed information on subjective phenomena was not developed until Lindsley and Leary devised the "experiential typewriter." This apparatus consisted of a 20-key typewriter connected to a recording instrument. The keys served to code various subjective states, including modes of perception, internal images, external images, images seen with the eyes closed and with the eyes open, hallucinations, colors and so on. Training consisted of having the subjects memorize the categories and the corresponding keys. When a subject felt a bodily sensation such as "pain," he pressed a specific key to signify the event. A hallucination with oscillating colors could be signified by pressing a different key.

In tests with the hallucinogens LSD and dimethyltryptamine Leary found that the muscular discoordination associated with those drugs interfered with pressing the keys. The problem could have been avoided with lower doses, and the key press could have been replaced by a verbal report. (Leary had found that verbal reporting was not disrupted by the drugs.) Therefore we decided to develop a verbal code for reporting drug-induced hallucinations.

On the basis of the previous results we constructed a list of eight forms (random, line, curve, web, lattice, tunnel, spiral and kaleidoscope), eight colors (black, violet, blue, green, yellow, orange, red and white) and eight patterns of movement (aimless, vertical, horizontal, oblique, explosive, concentric, rotational and pulsating) for subjects to employ in describing visual imagery. We then selected a group of subjects and trained them with slides illustrating the different categories. For example, in training related to the tunnel form we showed hundreds of different slides of tunnels so that the subjects would have a broad concept of the tunnel form. In this way new instances of the form, which might not have been perceived before, could be appropriately classified on the basis of common features. The subjects were trained to recognize all three categories (form, color and movement) in displays projected for eight milliseconds, with a one-second pause between displays. Our aim in making the displays brief was to simulate the rapid changes of imagery in hallucinations.

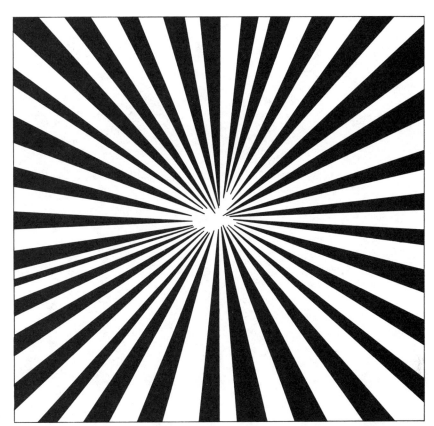

WHITE LIGHT seen during the early stages of intoxication with a hallucinogenic drug is portrayed. The visual imagery is reported to explode from the center to the periphery. Pattern appears initially in black and white, but bright colors may develop as the experience progresses.

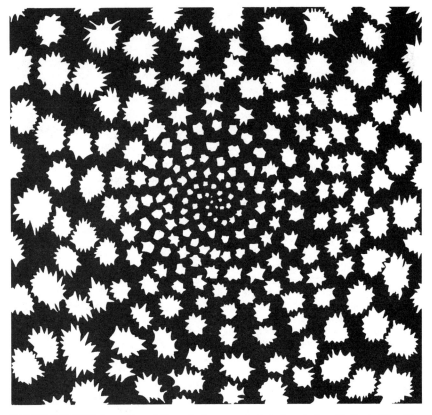

SPIRAL TUNNEL is another of the early form constants in drug-induced hallucination. The main patterns of movement accompanying the form are reported as pulsation and rotation.

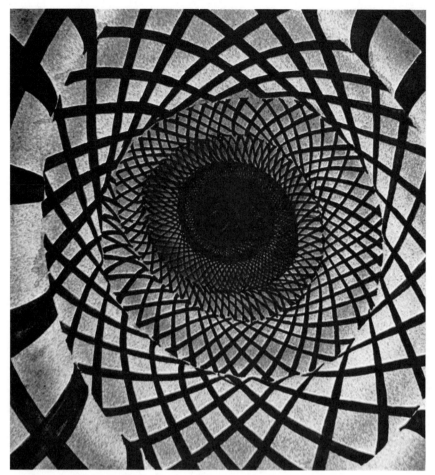

LATTICE-TUNNEL FORM CONSTANT is depicted in a painting made to show a pattern that is often reported during the early stages of intoxication from marihuana and tetrahydrocannabinol (the active principle of marihuana). It is possible that the blue color is related to the initial lowering of the body temperature and to the absorption of blue light by hemoglobin in "floater" cells in the retina. Colors tend to become red with time and with increasing dosage.

All the subjects, including some who were untrained so· that we could see if their reports of visual experiences were comparable to those of the trained subjects, then participated in a series of weekly test sessions in each of which they received either a hallucinogen, a stimulant, a depressant or a placebo. No subject knew what he was receiving. Both high and low doses were tested. The subjects were tested in the light-proof chamber I have mentioned. All the subjects were instructed to report what they "saw" with their eyes open, but the trained subjects were restricted to the descriptive code. In the middle of the session the trained subjects were tested with slides of real images to ensure that the drugs and dosages were not impairing the skills they had acquired in training. (We found no indication of impairment.)

The results were intriguing. We found that the trained subjects could keep abreast of the rapid flow of imagery and could readily classify most of the images into the categories of the reporting code. These subjects averaged 20 re-ports per minute; the untrained subjects reported only about five times per minute. (The duration of a typical session was six hours.)

The imagery associated with placebos, the stimulant *d*-amphetamine and the depressant phenobarbital was described as black-and-white random forms moving about aimlessly. The hallucinogens tetrahydrocannabinol, psilocybin, LSD and mescaline induced dramatic changes. Here the forms became less random and more organized and geometric as the experience progressed. The black-and-white images began to take on blue hues, and movement became more organized and pulsating. At 30 minutes after the administration of the drug the subjects reported a significant increase in lattice and tunnel forms and a slight increase in kaleidoscopic forms. By 90 and 120 minutes most forms were lattice-tunnels. Concomitantly the colors shifted to red, orange and yellow. Movement continued to be pulsating but became more organized, with explosive and rotational patterns.

Complex imagery usually did not appear until well after the shift to the lat-tice-tunnel forms was reported. Thereafter complex forms constituted from 43 to 75 percent of the forms reported by trained subjects who had received hallucinogens. The complex images first appeared in the reports as overlying the lattice-tunnels and situated on the periphery of those images.

Common complex images included childhood memories and scenes associated with strong emotional experiences that the subjects had undergone. These hallucinatory images were more than pictorial replicas; many of them were elaborated and embellished into fantastic scenes. This constructive aspect of imagery can be illustrated by a simple exercise. Recall the last time you went swimming in the ocean. Now ask yourself if this memory includes a picture of yourself running along the beach or moving about in the water. Such a picture is obviously fictitious, since you could not have been looking at yourself, but images in the memory often include fleeting pictures of this kind. Our subjects often reported equally improbable images, such as aerial perspectives and underwater views.

It has not been established where such constructions arise, but contributions are probably made in the encoding, storage and retrieval stages of the memory process. Much of the content of complex imagery can also be influenced by environmental stimuli. Since our subjects were in an isolated chamber, most of their images came from their memory. Occasionally, however, we escorted the subjects (at the peak of the hallucinatory experience) to a botanical garden. There they wore goggles through which they could not see, lay on the grass and reported what they "saw" with their eyes open. At these times the imagery from memory was reduced significantly, and reports of birds, airplanes, trees and so on increased. In other experiments we have shaped and guided drug-induced imagery by giving the subjects suggestive words or music. Nevertheless, even these primed complex images were usually reported as appearing in lattice-tunnel arrangements and moving in explosive or rotational configurations.

During the peak hallucinatory periods the subjects frequently described themselves as having become part of the imagery. At such times they stopped using similes in their reports and asserted that the images were real. This point marked the transition from pseudohallucination to true hallucination. Highly creative and fantastic combinations of imagery were reported, sometimes with as many as 10 changes of image per second. The subjects frequently reported feeling dissociated from their bodies.

The remarkable constancies of drug-induced hallucinations lead naturally to an inquiry into how universal they may be. Some of them are strikingly similar to the primordial or archetypal forms (such as the mandala, the mystic symbol of the universe employed in Hinduism and Buddhism as an aid to meditation) that the psychoanalyst C. G. Jung described as part of man's collective unconscious. Moreover, as many anthropologists have noted, the hallucinogen-inspired art of many primitive peoples often contains constants of form, color and movement.

We examined this phenomenon by traveling to the Sierra Madre of Mexico to study a group of Huichol Indians who take peyote. They have remained relatively isolated since Aztec times. We interviewed them during their peyote ceremonies, eliciting reports on their visual imagery. The images proved to be virtually identical to the symmetrical, repeat-

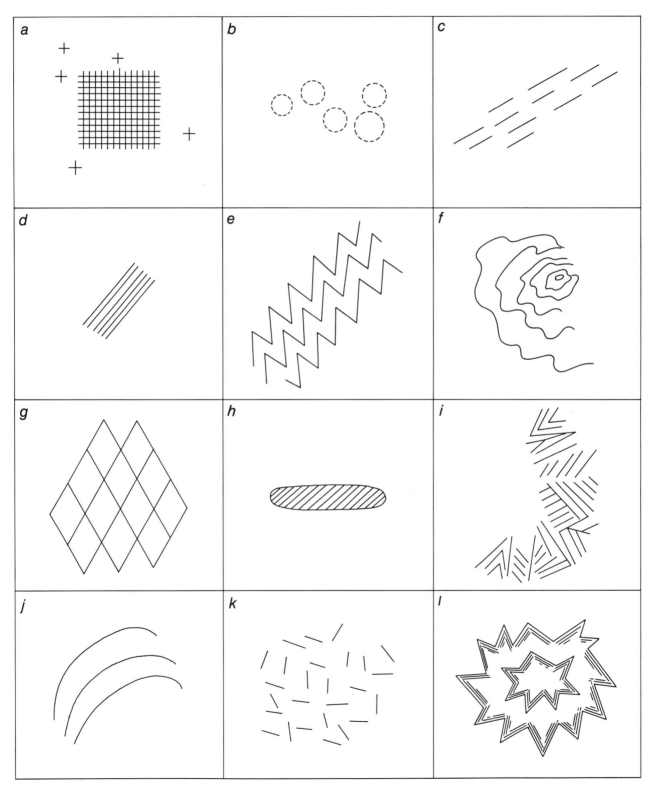

VISUAL HALLUCINATIONS seen during controlled intoxication with cocaine were drawn by people who served as subjects in the author's experiments. The patterns were usually seen with the eyes open in a dark room; they appeared as transitory black-and-white spots in the periphery of the visual field. Patterns c, e, f, g, i, k and l are virtually identical to the patterns seen in the hallucinations accompanying migraine attacks. Indeed, pattern l is the "fortification illusion" that is frequently reported by people who are suffering migraine headaches.

It looks like several different whirlpools, with lots of spirals divided up into checks. It's pretty black. There's purple and green glowing areas in the middle of the spirals, kind of clouds around. There are lines going from top to bottom, kind of a grid, but the lines squiggle around. There's odd shapes, but still lots of right angles in them. Seems really bright.... There's like an explosion, yellow in the middle, like a volcano gushing out lava, yellow, glowing. There's a black square with yellow light coming behind it. There's a regular pattern superimposed on everything, lots of curlicues, with dots in the middle. Lot of little paisley things that fill up the spaces between the patterns of triangles, squares, or crown-shaped things. And there's a little white star that floats around the picture and sometimes goes behind what's on the screen and illuminates from behind.

Now there's a kind of landscape. Very flat, flat country. The picture is very narrow. In the middle part a tree at the left and then flat with green grass and blue sky above. There are orange dots, oranges hanging all over, in the sky, on the tree, on the ground. A bicycle! Oh, my! It's headed down, not horizontal, like someone's holding it up on end.... There's a checkerboard superimposed on everything, like the flags they wave at the races.

I can see the street out there.... Well, it's old--golly--interesting! It's like in the forties, I guess, or maybe the fifties.... And there are people riding their bicycles, and there are, like, boys, in plaid vests and those funny kind of hats.... I was at the side walking on the sidewalk, so it wasn't like I was in the middle of the street and (laughter) you can't laugh very long in the middle of the street in the city, so that image kind of went away (laughter).

PARTIAL TRANSCRIPT of the remarks made by a subject who had taken 20 milligrams of the hallucinogen psilocybin shows an increasing complexity of imagery. The first paragraph is from an initial segment of the experience, which began about 25 minutes after the subject had taken the drug. The simple geometric forms are supplemented several minutes later (*second paragraph*) by complex images. They are later replaced (*third paragraph*) by dreamlike scenes.

ing patterns found in Huichol weaving and art.

In attempting to explain the origin of the simple hallucinatory constants a number of investigators have described them as the product of events within the eye resulting from the visualization of certain structures when light strikes the eye in a particular way. For example, horizontal bands are said to be due to folds in the corneal epithelium that change with motion of the eyelid, and a black lacework seen against a red background is attributed to shadows cast on the rods and cones by blood vessels of the retina.

Since such causes require light, they cannot have figured prominently in our experiments, which were conducted in darkness. Light is not necessary, however, for the production of phosphenes, which are visual sensations arising from the discharge of neurons in structures of the eye. Phosphenes can include spots, disks, concentric arcs or circles and checkerboard patterns.

The constants are also highly similar to the patterns found in hallucinations accompanying migraine attacks. Migraine patterns include lines, grids, concentric circles and the "fortification illusion," which is a horseshoe-shaped area consisting of bright zigzag lines appearing at an expanding outer edge. Migraine hallucinations can also be brightly colored and explosive and can include complex images of people and objects. The most plausible explanation of migraine phenomena is that they reflect the electrical excitation of organized groups of cells in the visual cortex of the brain. Indeed, the work of Wilder Penfield and his colleagues at McGill University has shown that the direct electrical stimulation of the visual cortex or the temporal lobes gives rise to moving colored lights, geometric forms, stars and lines.

Most of the investigators undertaking to explain complex hallucinatory imagery have described the images as the result of an excitation of the central nervous system. As early as 1845 Moreau was maintaining that hallucinations resulted from cerebral excitation that enabled thoughts and memories to become transformed into sensory impressions. Recent electrophysiological research has confirmed that hallucinations are directly related to states of excitation and arousal of the central nervous system, which are coupled with a functional disorganization of the part of the brain that regulates incoming stimuli. Behaviorally the result is an impairment of the discrimination normally based on external stimuli and a preoccupation with internal imagery.

This hallucinatory process has been described by such terms as "memory flashback" and "involuntary reminiscence." Certain psychoanalysts have postulated that it is the result of a general regression to primitive or childlike thinking, coupled with the emergence of repressed information and memories. Students of psychedelic phenomena have postulated that hallucinogens release normally suppressed information and memories.

Perhaps the most integrated explanation has been provided by the perceptual-release theory of hallucinations, which was formulated by the British neurologist Hughlings Jackson in 1931. As recently brought up to date by Louis Jolyon West of UCLA, the hypothesis assumes that normal memories are suppressed by a mechanism that acts as a gate to the flow of information from the outside. An input of new information inhibits the emergence and awareness of previous perceptions and processed information. If the input is decreased or impaired while awareness remains, such perceptions are released and may be dynamically organized and experienced as hallucinations, dreams or fantasies.

West has offered an analogy to illustrate the process. Picture a man in his living room, standing at a closed window opposite his fireplace and looking out at the sunset. He is absorbed by the view of the outside world and does not visualize the interior of the room. As darkness falls outside, however, the images of the objects in the room behind him can be seen reflected dimly in the window. With the deepening of darkness the fire in the fireplace illuminates the room, and the man now sees a vivid reflection of the room, which appears to be outside the window. As the analogy is applied to the perceptual-release hypothesis, the daylight (the sensory input) is reduced while the interior illumination (the general level of arousal of the central nervous system) remains bright, so that images originating within the rooms of the brain may be perceived as though they came from outside the windows of the senses.

Through such research and hypotheses we have begun to understand the nature of hallucinations as stored images in the brain. Like a mirage that shows a magnificent city, the images of hallucinations are actually reflected images of real objects located elsewhere. The city is no less intriguing and no less worthy of study because it is not where we think it is. Further experiments will help localize it.

THE AUTHORS

JOSEPH S. LEVINE and EDWARD F. MAC-NICHOL, JR. ("Color Vision in Fishes") are sensory physiologists with a special interest in aquatic animals. Levine is assistant professor of biology at Boston College and a research associate at the Marine Biological Laboratory in Woods Hole, Mass. He was graduated from Tufts University in 1973 and went on to obtain a master's degree at Boston University in 1976, writing his thesis on the aquaculture of lobsters. He received his Ph.D. in biology from Harvard University in 1980. MacNichol is director of the laboratory of sensory physiology at Woods Hole and professor of physiology at Boston University School of Medicine. After getting an undergraduate degree at Princeton University in 1941 he went to the Radiation Laboratory of the Massachusetts Institute of Technology. He received his Ph.D. from Johns Hopkins University in 1952. He has long been interested in the measurement of electrical activity in individual nerve cells. His initial studies included some of the first intracellular recordings from the photoreceptor cells of the lateral eye of the horseshoe crab. MacNichol left Johns Hopkins in 1968 to become director of the National Institute of Neurological Diseases and Stroke, a position he held until 1973. For part of that time he was also the acting director of the National Eye Institute.

G. ADRIAN HORRIDGE ("The Compound Eye of Insects") is a professor in the department of zoology at the University of Cambridge. Born in England, he received his undergraduate and graduate education at Cambridge, studying subjects ranging from jellyfish nerve networks to the coral reefs of the Red Sea to Persian carpets. His first job was at the Royal Aircraft Establishment at Farnborough, where he worked on the design of engineering structures made with composite materials. From there he went to St. Andrew's University, where he later became director of the Gatty Marine Laboratory. In 1969 Horridge went to the Australian National University in Canberra, where he founded the department of neurobiology. He returned to Cambridge in 1977. His principal avocation

is the study of Indonesian boatbuilding at the shipyards where these traditional sailing vessels are still being built. "This interest has taken me to remote parts of Java, Madura, Bali, Timor, the Moluccas and Celebes and to equally inaccessible libraries and collections," he writes.

ERIC A. NEWMAN and PETER H. HARTLINE ("The Infrared 'Vision' of Snakes") are respectively assistant scientist and associate scientist at the Eye Research Institute of the Retina Foundation in Boston. They have collaborated in work on the infrared sense of snakes since 1978. Newman obtained his bachelor's, master's and doctoral degrees from the Massachusetts Institute of Technology; his Ph.D., granted in 1977, is in biology. Hartline received his undergraduate education at Swarthmore College. He earned a master's degree at Harvard University and, in 1969, a Ph.D. in neuroscience from the University of California at San Diego. From 1969 to 1974 he was assistant research scientist at the University of California at San Diego. In 1974 he went to the University of Illinois at Urbana-Champaign, and in 1977 he moved to the Eye Research Institute.

DAVID H. HUBEL and TORSTEN N. WIESEL ("Brain Mechanisms of Vision") have collaborated on studies of the mammalian visual system for nearly 20 years. Wiesel is Vincent and Brooke Astor Professor and head of the laboratory of neurobiology at the Rockefeller University. Born in Sweden, he obtained his M.D. in 1954 at the Karolinska Institute in Stockholm. After a year as an instructor of physiology there he came to the U.S. to join the faculty of the Johns Hopkins University School of Medicine. He moved to the Harvard Medical School in 1959.

OLGA EIZNER FAVREAU and MICHAEL C. CORBALLIS ("Negative Aftereffects in Visual Perception") are respectively assistant professor of psychology at the University of Montreal and professor of psychology at McGill University. Favreau was born and educated in Montreal and earned her Ph.D. at McGill in 1973. She joined the faculty at Montreal in 1974. Her work in visual perception grew out of her interests in psychology and in the visual arts. She is also concerned with the position of women in society, which has led her to look into research on differences in abilities according to sex. She served a one-year term as a member of the Canadian Psychological Association's Task Force on the Status of Women in Psychology, where she did a survey of bias in research on sex differences. Corballis was born in New Zealand but is now a Canadian citizen. After being graduated from Victoria University College in New Zealand in 1959 with a master's degree in mathematics he switched to psychology, obtaining a master's in 1962 from the University of Auckland. Three years later he received his Ph.D. in psychology from McGill. After a brief period as a lecturer in psychology at Auckland he returned to McGill as a member of the faculty. Corballis is interested in most aspects of human experimental psychology, and this year he and Ivan L. Beale published a book titled *The Psychology of Left and Right*. He writes: "My wife and I both make stoneware pottery, she with greater expertise than I, and I can beat Olga Favreau at squash."

ROBERT SEKULER and EUGENE LEVINSON ("The Perception of Moving Targets") are at Northwestern University, where Sekuler is professor and chairman of the department of psychology and Levinson is a postdoctoral fellow and visiting scholar in the university's Biomedical Engineering Center. Sekular is a graduate of Brandeis University and holds a Ph.D. from Brown University. He joined the faculty at Northwestern in 1965, after having spent a postdoctoral year at the Massachusetts Institute of Technology. He describes himself as a "fanatical sailor" who is "also active in the Greater Chicago branch of the American Begonia Society." His collaboration with Levinson on a number of projects in visual perception began in 1971, when Levinson took an undergraduate course on perception taught by Sekuler. Levinson went on to do graduate work at Dalhousie University, returning to earn his Ph.D. from Northwestern in 1976. His current research interests are in the area of retinal physiology and pharmacology.

JEREMY M. WOLFE ("Hidden Visual Processes") teaches introductory psychology at the Massachusetts Institute of Technology and does research in the institute's Center for Cognitive Science. Born in London, he was graduated summa cum laude from Princeton University in 1977. He did his graduate work on binocular vision with Richard Held at M.I.T, getting his Ph.D. in 1981. He writes: "In high school I thought I would become a lawyer or perhaps a rabbi, but I was 'converted' to the experimental psychology of vision by a summer job at Bell Laboratories. I spent my time sitting in a dark room looking at barely visi-

ble flashes of colored light and came out determined to do the same to other people." When Wolfe is not working in the classroom or the laboratory, he adds, "I live in Newton, Mass., with one wife, two cats (one without a tail) and one six-foot Burmese python."

GAETANO KANIZSA ("Subjective Contours") is professor of psychology at the University of Trieste. He received his doctorate in psychology from the University of Padua, where, he notes, he was "imbued with the European Gestalt tradition." Since then he has dedicated himself "to the phenomenology of visual perception and thought processes." He carried on his work in Florence and Milan before returning to his native city of Trieste in 1953 to take up his present post. In addition to his psychological research he is also "interested in the relation between science and the visual arts" and is "actively engaged in painting."

BARBARA GILLAM ("Geometrical Illusions") teaches and does research in visual perception and binocular vision at the College of Optometry of the State University of New York. Born in Australia, she studied psychology as an undergraduate at the University of Sydney and went on to obtain a Ph.D. for her work on binocular vision from the Australian National University. After a few years on the faculty of the University of Reading in England, she immigrated to the U.S. in 1967. Gillam writes: "I first became interested in illusions because I do not have a car and I frequently travel on the New York subway system and on buses. I find that doodling illusion figures with paper and pencil is much less attention-getting than trying out ideas in binocular vision, which involves frequently opening and closing one eye."

DONALD D. HOFFMAN ("The Interpretation of Visual Illusions") is assistant professor of cognitive science and computer science at the University of California at Irvine. He got a B.A. in 1978 from the University of California at Los Angeles before going on to earn his Ph.D. in computational psychology in 1983 from the Massachusetts Institute of Technology.

LYNN A. COOPER and ROGER N. SHEPARD ("Turning Something Over in the Mind") are experimental psychologists who have collaborated extensively on the study of mental images. Cooper is associate professor of psychology at the University of Pittsburgh and senior scientist at its Learning Research and Development Center and its Center for the Philosophy of Science. She went to the University of Michigan as an undergraduate and got her Ph.D. from Stanford University in 1973. Cooper has won the American Psychologist Association's Distinguished Scientific Award for an Early Career Contribution to Psychology. Shepard is professor of psychology at Stanford. He earned his undergraduate degree at Stanford in 1951 and his Ph.D. from Yale University in 1955. In 1968 he returned to Stanford as a member of the faculty. He has received a number of awards and fellowships including the Distinguished Scientific Contribution Award of the American Psychological Association, and is a member of the National Academy of Sciences. Shepard and Cooper first worked together when she was a graduate student at Stanford; the book *Mental Images and Their Transformations* (The MIT Press/Bradford Books, 1982), of which they are coauthors, surveys their ensuing research.

RONALD K. SIEGEL ("Hallucinations") is associate research psychologist in the Department of Psychiatry and Biobehavioral Sciences and also adjunct associate professor of psychology at the University of California at Los Angeles. He did his undergraduate work at Brandeis University in 1970. Before joining the UCLA faculty he spent two years as a postdoctoral fellow in pharmacology at the Albert Einstein College of Medicine in New York.

BIBLIOGRAPHY

I EYES

1. Color Vision in Fishes

VISION IN FISHES. Edited by M. A. Ali. Plenum Press, 1975.

THE EVOLUTION OF PHOTOPIC VISUAL PIGMENTS IN FISHES: PART III, W. N. McFarland and F. W. Munz in *Vision Research*, Vol. 15, No. 10, pages 1071–1080; October, 1975.

THE ECOLOGY OF VISION, J. N. Lythgoe. Oxford University Press, 1979.

2. The Compound Eye of Insects

THE SIZE OF OMMATIDIA IN APPOSITION EYES. Horace B. Barlow in *The Journal of Experimental Biology*, Vol. 29, No. 4, pages 667–674; December, 1952.

PHYSICAL ASPECTS OF THE SENSE ORGANS. Hl. de Vries in *Progress in Biophysics and Biophysical Chemistry*, Vol. 6, pages 208–264; 1956.

THE VISUAL SYSTEM OF INSECTS. Timothy H. Goldsmith and Gary D. Bernard in *The Physiology of Insects: Vol. II*, edited by Morris Rockstein. Academic Press, Inc., 1974.

THE COMPOUND EYE AND VISION OF INSECTS. Edited by G. Adrian Horridge. Oxford University Press, 1975.

PHOTORECEPTOR OPTICS. Edited by A. W. Snyder and R. Menzel. Springer-Verlag, 1975.

3. The Infrared "Vision" of Snakes

PROPERTIES OF AN INFRA-RED RECEPTOR. T. H. Bullock and F. P. J. Diecke, in *the Journal of Physiology*, Vol. 134, pages 47–87; October, 1956.

RATTLESNAKES: THEIR HABITS, LIFE HISTORIES AND INFLUENCE OF MANKIND. Lawrence M. Klauber. The University of California Press, 2d ed., 1972.

THERMORECEPTORS IN SNAKES. P. H. Hartline in *Handbook of Sensory Physiology*, Vol. III/3: *Electroreceptors and Other Specialized Receptors in Lower Vertebrates*, Springer-Verlag, 1974.

MERGING OF MODALITIES IN THE OPTIC TECTUM: INFRARED AND VISUAL INTEGRATION IN RATTLESNAKES. P. H. Hartline, L. Kass, and M. S. Loop, in *Science*, vol. 199, pages 1225–1229; March 17, 1978.

INTEGRATION OF VISUAL AND INFRARED INFORMATION IN BIMODAL NEURONS OF THE RATTLESNAKE OPTIC TECTUM. E. A. Newman and P. H. Hartline, in *Science*, vol. 213, pages 789–791; August 14, 1981.

II PATHWAYS TO THE MIND'S EYE

4. Brain Mechanisms of Vision

MODALITY AND TOPOGRAPHIC PROPERTIES OF SINGLE NEURONS OF CAT'S SOMATIC SENSORY CORTEX. V. B. Mountcastle in *The Journal of Neurophysiology*, Vol. 20, No. 4, pages 408–434; July, 1957.

RECEPTIVE FIELDS AND FUNCTIONAL ARCHITECTURE OF MONKEY STRIATE CORTEX. D. H. Hubel and T. N. Wiesel in *The Journal of Physiology*, Vol. 195, No. 2, pages 215–244; November, 1968.

FERRIER LECTURE: FUNCTIONAL ARCHITECTURE OF MACAQUE MONKEY VISUAL CORTEX. D. H. Hubel and T. N. Wiesel in *Proceedings of the Royal Society of London, Series B*, Vol. 198, pages 1–59; 1977.

ANATOMICAL DEMONSTRATION OF ORIENTATION COLUMNS IN MACAQUE MONKEY. David H. Hubel, Torsten N. Wiesel and Michael P. Stryker in *The Journal of Comparative Neurology*, Vol. 177, No. 3, pages 361–379; February 1, 1978.

5.   Negative Aftereffects in Visual Perception

COMPARISON OF NORMALIZATION THEORY AND NEURAL ENHANCEMENT EXPLANATION OF NEGATIVE AFTEREFFECTS. Ray Over in *Psychological Bulletin*, Vol. 75, No. 4, pages 225–243; April, 1971.

HANDBOOK OF PERCEPTION, VOL. I: HISTORICAL AND PHILOSOPHICAL ROOTS OF PERCEPTION. Edited by Edward C. Carterette and Morton P. Friedman. Academic Press, 1973.

SIGHT AND MIND: AN INTRODUCTION TO VISUAL PERCEPTION. Lloyd Kaufman, Oxford University Press, 1974.

WHAT DOES VISUAL PERCEPTION TELL US ABOUT VISUAL CODING? Stuart M. Anstis in *Handbook of Psychobiology*, edited by Michael S. Gazzaniga and Colin Blakemore. Academic Press, 1975.

MCCOLLOUGH EFFECTS: EXPERIMENTAL FINDINGS AND THEORETICAL ACCOUNTS. D. Showko, B. N. Timeny, T. A. Gentry and R. B. Morant in *Psychological Bulletin*, Vol. 82, No. 4, pages 479–510; July, 1975.

6.   The Perception of Moving Targets

INHIBITION AND DISINHIBITION OF DIRECTION-SPECIFIC MECHANISMS IN HUMAN VISION. Eugene Levinson and Robert Sekuler in *Nature*, Vol. 254, No. 5502, pages 692–694; April 24, 1975.

MOVING VISUAL PHANTOMS: A NEW CONTOUR COMPLETION EFFECT. Paul Tynan and Robert Sekuler in *Science*, Vol. 188, No. 4191, pages 951–952; May 30, 1975.

THE INDEPENDENCE OF CHANNELS IN HUMAN VISION SELECTIVE FOR DIRECTION OF MOVEMENT. Eugene Levinson and Robert Sekular in *The Journal of Physiology*, Vol. 250, No. 2, pages 347–366; September, 1975.

7.   Hidden Visual Processes

EYE TORSION AND VISUAL TILT ARE MEDIATED BY DIFFERENT BINOCULAR PROCESSES. Jeremy M. Wolfe and Richard Held in *Vision Research*, Vol. 19, No. 8, pages 917–920; 1979.

CYCLOPEAN STIMULATION CAN INFLUENCE SENSATIONS OF SELF-MOTION IN NORMAL AND STEREOBLIND SUBJECTS. Jeremy M. Wolfe and Richard Held in *Perception and Psychophysics*, Vol. 28, No. 2, pages 139–142; 1980.

INTEROCULAR TRANSFER OF VISUAL AFTEREFFECTS. R. Blake, R. Overton and S. Lema-Stern in *Journal of Experimental Psychology: HPP*, Vol. 7, pages 367–381; 1981.

IS ACCOMMODATION COLORBLIND? FOCUSING CHROMATIC CONTOURS. Jeremy M. Wolfe and D. Alfred Owens in *Perception*, Vol. 10, pages 53–62; 1981.

A PURELY BINOCULAR MECHANISM IN HUMAN VISION. Jeremy M. Wolfe and Richard Held in *Vision Research*, Vol. 21, No. 12, pages 1755–1759; 1981.

III   IN THE MIND'S EYE

8.   Subjective Contours

STEREOPSIS AND ANOMALOUS CONTOUR. R. B. Lawson and W. L. Gulick in *Vision Research*, Vol. 7, pages 271–297; March, 1967.

SELECTIVE HISTORY OF THEORIES OF VISUAL PERCEPTION: 1650–1950. Nicholas Pastore. Oxford University Press, 1971.

UNTERSUCHUNGEN ZUM PROBLEM VIRTUELLER KONTUREN IN DER VISUELLEN WAHRNEHMUNG. Michael Stadler and Jürgen Dieker in *Zeitschrift für experimentelle und angewandte Psychologie*, Vol. 19, No. 2, pages 325–350; 1972.

SUBJECTIVE CONTOURS AND APPARENT DEPTH. Stanley Coren in *Psychological Review*, Vol. 79, No. 4, pages 359–367; July, 1972.

COGNITIVE CONTOURS. R. L. Gregory in *Nature*, Vol. 238, No. 5358, pages 51–52; July 7, 1972.

CONTOURS WITHOUT GRADIENTS OR COGNITIVE CONTOURS? Gaetano Kanizsa in *Italian Journal of Psychology*, Vol. 1, No. 1, pages 93–112; April, 1974.

9.   Geometrical Illusions

A DEPTH PROCESSING THEORY OF THE POGGENDORFF ILLUSION. B. Gillam in *Perception and Psychophysics*, Vol. 10, No. 4A, pages 211–216; 1971.

THE PSYCHOLOGY OF VISUAL ILLUSION, J. O. Robinson. Hutchinson University Library, 1972.

ILLUSION IN NATURE AND ART. Edited By R. L. Gregory and E. H. Gombrich. Charles Scribner's Sons, 1973.

SEEING IS DECEIVING: THE PSYCHOLOGY OF VISUAL ILLUSIONS. Stanley Coren and Joan S. Girgus. Lawrence Erlbaum Associates, 1978.

10.   The Interpretation of Visual Illusions

DIFFERENTIAL GEOMETRY OF CURVES AND SURFACES. Manfredo P. do Carmo. Prentice-Hall, Inc., 1976.

VISION: A COMPUTATIONAL INVESTIGATION INTO THE HUMAN REPRESENTAITON AND PROCESSING OF VISUAL INFORMATION. David Marr. W. H. Freeman and Company, 1982.

THE MODULARITY OF MIND. Jerry Fodor. The MIT Press, 1983.

11. Turning Something Over in the Mind

MENTAL ROTATION OF THREE-DIMENSIONAL OBJECTS. R. N. Shepard and J. Metzler in *Science*, Vol. 171, No. 3972, pages 701–703; February 19, 1971.

MENTAL ROTATION OF RANDOM TWO-DIMENSIONAL SHAPES. Lynn A. Cooper in *Cognitive Psychology*, Vol. 7, No. 1, pages 20–43; January, 1975.

PERCEPTION. Julian E. Hochberg. Prentice-Hall, Inc., 1978.

ECOLOGICAL CONSTRAINTS ON INTERNAL REPRESENTATION: RESORT KINEMATICS OF PERCEIVING, IMAGINING, THINKING AND DREAMING. R. N. Shepard in *Psychological Review*, Vol. 91, No. 4, pages 417–447; October, 1984.

12. Hallucinations

MESCAL AND MECHANISMS OF HALLUCINATIONS. Heinrich Klüver. The University of Chicago Press, 1966.

HASHISH AND MENTAL ILLNESS. J. J. Moreau. Raven Press, 1973.

HALLUCINATIONS: BEHAVIOR, EXPERIENCE AND THEORY. Edited by Ronald K. Siegel and Louis Jolyon West. John Wiley & Sons, Inc., 1975.

INDEX